yoga
TO GO

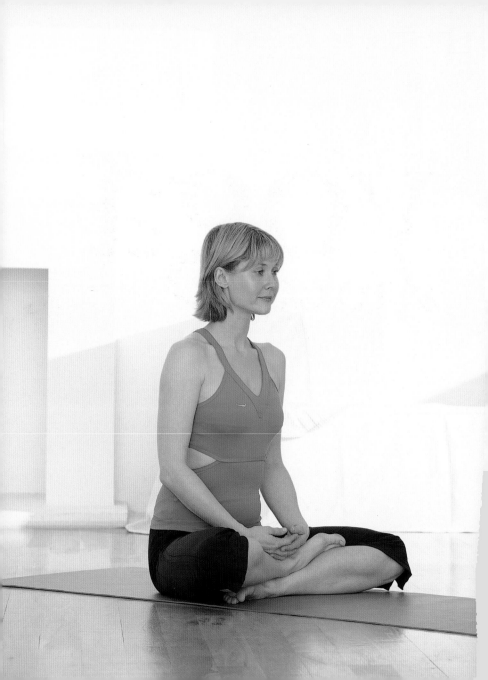

yoga
TO GO

Stella Weller

An Hachette Livre UK Company

First published in Great Britain in 2008 by
Gaia Books, a division of Octopus Publishing Group Ltd
2–4 Heron Quays, London E14 4JP
www.octopusbooks.co.uk

This material was previously published as *A Gaia Busy Person's Guide: Yoga*

ISBN: 978-1-85675-295-4

A CIP catalogue record for this book is available from the British Library

Printed and bound in China

10 9 8 7 6 5 4 3 2 1

Cautionary note:
All reasonable care has been taken in the preparation of this book, but the information it contains is not meant to take the place of medical care under the direct supervision of a doctor. Before making any changes in your health regime, always consult a doctor. While all the therapies detailed in this book are completely safe if done correctly, you must seek professional advice if you are in any doubt about any medical condition. Any application of the ideas and information contained in this book is at the reader's sole discretion and risk.

Direction Patrick Nugent
Production Louise Hall
Editors Fiona Biggs, Kelly Thomson
Design Phil Gamble
Photography Ruth Jenkinson

Contents

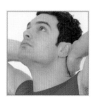

Using this book

A good guide shows you the way as you explore new terrain, or helps you to rediscover territory with which you may once have been familiar. This book is such a guide, providing direction, encouragement, and wise counsel along the path of your yoga journey. It has been designed for you, the busy person, to show you how to integrate this time-honoured system of health promotion and personal growth into your daily life. Even if you can spare no more than five minutes a day for exercising, you can combine the exercises to create a workout to suit your own special needs. Before you begin, though, check with your doctor and read the information in Chapter One thoroughly, even if yoga is not new to you. It is here that you will learn what yoga is and is not, and what guidelines you should follow for safe, effective practice. You will learn what yoga comprises and how it works to help you to cope in an increasingly stressful world. You will read about the advantages to be derived from practising in the morning and those to expect from evening practice, and you will find out about various places where you can safely do the exercises. You will discover how you can incorporate many of the exercises into your work day, no matter what your job is, to reap the cumulative benefits of this superb health-care system.

Chapter Two offers safe, simple, enjoyable warm-up exercises that will wake you up gently and generate energy for the day. You will also learn essential cooling-down techniques.

Chapter Three is devoted to travelling. Here you will find techniques that you can practise safely even while

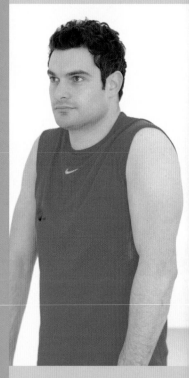

FINDING TIME FOR YOGA
Shoulder rotation is a simple exercise that you can do in just a few seconds during the working day. Rotating your shoulders a few times will discourage tension build-up and joint stiffness (see p.23).

on the road, to help in coping with stressful traffic situations. Suggestions are also given for incorporating exercises in Chapter Two to help to make travelling the pleasant experience it could be, and to avoid the anxiety, circulation problems, and jet lag with which frequent flyers are often familiar.

Staying calm under pressure, combating fatigue, and boosting energy and productivity at work are the topics addressed in Chapter Four, which provides simple but effective techniques that you can weave into the fabric of your daily schedule, to help you to act calmly rather than react impulsively. Suggestions are also given for preventing conditions such as backache, neck pain, eye strain, and carpal tunnel syndrome, which have become almost epidemic in today's fast-moving, highly competitive world.

Returning home after the day's activities often presents another set of challenges. Chapter Five offers a number of "tools" to help you to unwind and to savour the sanctuary of a warm, secure environment where you can recharge yourself and feel at peace. Among these are breathing techniques that take advantage of one of our most under-utilized natural resources (the breath), and exercises in which you apply the principles of meditation to activities of choice, to induce the state that doctors describe as "restful alertness". You will also find out how to promote sound, refreshing sleep without the aid of medication. A specimen yoga programme, which you can tailor to suit your unique set of circumstances, is offered for your weekend enjoyment and relaxation.

HELPING HANDS
Tension can accumulate in the hands. Tightening and releasing the muscles of the fingers, hands, and arms several times a day will avert repetitive strain injury to the wrists (see also pp.24, 25, 106–7).

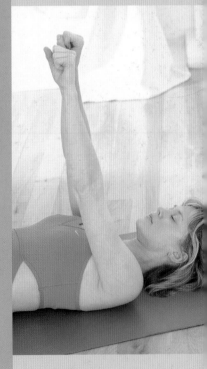

Introduction

Because yoga has its roots in the Hindu culture, some people are understandably nervous about practising it. They fear it may be incompatible with their religious beliefs. But this fear is unfounded. Yoga is non-sectarian and may be practised with complete confidence by anyone. If the word itself poses a problem, however, then think of it as a useful package containing safe, simple, effective stress-reduction techniques such as gentle stretching and breathing exercises, and relaxation, concentration, and meditation techniques.

There are many forms of yoga, but the one that has gained the most

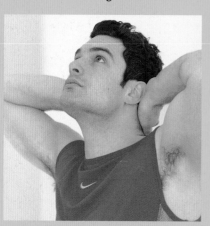

popularity, particularly in the West, is Hatha Yoga, or the yoga of health. Its primary goal is to prevent illness and maintain a harmonious body-mind equilibrium. If illness occurs, those who practise yoga regularly will regain health speedily through a balanced system of physical and mental exercises.

The physical exercises, called asanas or postures, benefit not only muscles and joints but also internal structures such as organs, nerves, and glands. In addition, they train and discipline the mind so as to improve concentration and coordination, and they are superb for preventing the build-up of tension that often leads to aches and pains, and that also sometimes causes inappropriate responses and poor impulse control. The exercises are, moreover, excellent for improving posture and carriage, thus enhancing self-esteem, on which our feelings of self-confidence depend.

The mental and breathing exercises (the latter are collectively called pranayama) are probably without match for combating stress, and the relaxation techniques are a very useful adjunct to treatments for disorders such as depression and high blood pressure.

Because yoga exercises encourage a full focusing on what is being done, they promote an ability to "tune in" to yourself, thus fostering the development of a keen sense of awareness which alerts you to the early warning signs of departures from good health. Regular practice will give you a strong sense of balance and wholeness, and of being at peace with yourself.

Yoga differs from many other types of exercise in that it engages the whole person. It requires your full attention during practice, so your mind and body work together to create psychological and physiological harmony.

Yoga, however, is not a "quick fix". Do not immediately expect dramatic results. These will be proportionate only to the effort you make. Integrating yoga exercises into activities of daily living, until they become almost second nature, is perhaps the best way of ensuring regularity of practice. In this way, you will not think of them as something to be gotten over and done with, but rather as a pleasurable and anticipated part of day-to-day living.

Yoga practice conditions the body and the mind to adapt to environmental influences, both external and internal.

Rather than just alleviating symptoms, the exercises address the less evident, but very important, underlying causes of certain states and conditions.

Yoga's stretching, strengthening, and meditative exercises are effective because they require full focus on the movements of the body parts involved, in synchronization with attentive respiration (breathing). The mind, discouraged from wandering toward unrelated matters, is kept centred, engendering feelings of being calmer and more organized.

The directing of the attention away from distracting or disturbing stimuli and concentrating it on one thing or activity at a time has a soothing, settling effect. Energy is consequently conserved rather than squandered.

Through the regular practice of the techniques done in this manner, you come to know your body, and you increasingly get in touch with your feelings in a more intimate way than through practising exercises in an automatic, repetitive fashion which allows the mind to drift randomly. This mindfulness is excellent for promoting calm and control, invaluable attributes for stress-proofing yourself.

CHAPTER ONE

Getting started

The word yoga comes from Sanskrit, the language of ancient India. It means union, integration, or wholeness. It is an approach to health that promotes the harmonious collaboration of the human being's three components: body, mind, and spirit.

Perhaps no other period in history has been as fast-paced as the present one. Every day we hurry to fulfil various family and social obligations and to participate in numerous other activities with seemingly unrealistic time constraints. Many people are expected to perform their jobs with the same speed and accuracy as machines. But although machines have become increasingly rapid, humans can work only at a human pace.

Attempts to accede to the demands of this new technology are made at tremendous cost, both financially and in terms of human suffering. Occupational illnesses such as lower back pain, eye strain, and hand and wrist disabilities are on the rise. The incidence of stress-related disorders such as arthritis, depression, and heart disease has increased. But our capacity for dealing with these disorders has not grown proportionately, and mainstream therapies for them do not always have the beneficial effects that we might hope for.

The answer to these problems lies not in exclusive dependence on outside agents such as drugs, but rather in exploring and utilizing our rich store of inner resources. We can tap into these through the regular practice of yoga, an age-old technology of physical and mental wholeness and personal growth, which requires no props or gadgets, no special clothing or equipment. Yoga now forms the basis of many respected health-promotion programmes and stress-reduction and healing regimens worldwide.

Introducing yoga

Yoga works to maintain health and harmony by encouraging the cultivation of sound psychological attitudes through mental exercises, and breathing and relaxation techniques. It also reconditions the nerve-muscle and nerve-gland systems to enable them to withstand high levels of stress and strain, by means of physical and breathing exercises.

BASIC GUIDELINES

What most characterizes yoga exercises and differentiates them from many other types of exercise is the attentiveness required while doing them. This makes them safe to do because you are promptly alerted to whether you are stretching, bending, or turning beyond the point of safety. Before attempting to do any of the exercises, however, check with your doctor. Be especially careful if you have a serious health problem, have had surgery of any kind, or are pregnant.

BEFORE YOU BEGIN

As a busy person, you will be fitting in the exercises wherever you conveniently can during the course of your day. You are also encouraged to try to set aside a longer period of time each week, for a more comprehensive yoga session. At such times, start with a few quiet moments to distance yourself mentally from everyday concerns or those that claim your attention at present. Close your eyes. Relax your jaw. Breathe slowly and smoothly. Relax your hands. Set the scene for the exercises you are about to do.

Begin with a few simple warm-ups, such as those offered in Chapter Two. At the end of your exercise session, cool down and recover appropriately. Most of the exercises in Chapter Two, done slowly, are also suitable for this purpose, and many yoga classes end with the pose of tranquillity (see Chapter 5, pp.102–7).

COMFORT AND SAFETY

Remove from your person any object that may cause pressure or injury, such as a tight belt or spectacles. Wear non-constricting clothing to permit ease of movement and breathing. If it is convenient and inconspicuous, loosen your tie or bra and remove your shoes. Emptying your bladder is an added comfort measure, if circumstances allow it.

If preparing for an exercise session of any length (half an hour or more), remember not to exercise within two hours of eating a heavy meal. This caution is particularly important if you have a history of angina (pain in the region of the heart). You may practise one hour after eating a light snack, or you may exercise after drinking a cup of tea or other non-alcoholic beverage.

If you plan to practise before breakfast, when your blood sugar level is low after a night without food, you may drink a glass of juice or eat something light, such as a slice of wholegrain bread. This is preferable to exercising on an empty stomach.

WHEN TO PRACTISE
Do appropriate exercises whenever you begin to feel tense, anxious, or tired, to prevent these states from reaching a level that is not conducive to calm, productivity, and general well-being. Exercising before you start your day's work can counteract morning stiffness and give you energy. Do try a combination of the exercises in Chapter Two whenever possible.

Exercising in the evening can relax you after a challenging day and induce that healthy tiredness that promotes sound, refreshing sleep. You may find a sequence of the exercises described in Chapter Five appropriate. Experiment to determine which times are best for you.

Look for opportunities throughout the day (and if you are a shift worker, during the evening or night) to incorporate appropriate techniques into your schedule. In my clinical practice I have often done this to give relief to tired legs, feet, and back.

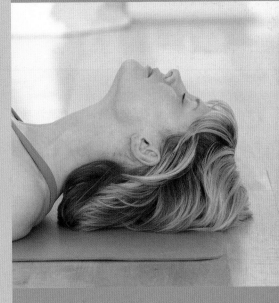

It is better to exercise for ten minutes every day than for half an hour only once a week. When re-starting after an illness or other interruption, do so gradually and patiently. Avoid trying to make up for lost time.

WHERE TO PRACTISE
One of the marvellous things about yoga is that you can practise it in a variety of places, indoors or outdoors, and you can even practise it in places where space is limited.

Moreover, you do not need to invest in any manufactured equipment: your body, your breath, and your attention are all that you require.

Ideally, the place where you practise your exercises should be quiet and well-ventilated. Distractions should be kept to a minimum. If practising at home, ask the family not to disturb you for the duration of your session.

The ground or floor on which you do the asanas should be smooth and level. A carpeted floor is suitable, or you can practise on a non-skid mat. A level grassy surface is also fine. The surface on which you exercise will be referred to as the "mat" in the exercise instructions throughout this book.

There are many opportunities for incorporating yoga exercises into daily activities. Suggestions are given alongside the instructions for many of the exercises. With practice, you will quickly build up your own repertoire of what to do and where to do it.

HOW TO PRACTISE
Practise each exercise slowly and mindfully, that is, with full attention to your movements. Synchronize these movements with slow, regular breathing through your nose (unless instructed otherwise), so that the inhaled air is warmed, moistened, and filtered before it reaches your lungs.

When you have completed a posture, hold it for a few seconds (increasing the duration as you become more practised and have the time), before resuming your starting position. Do not hold your breath during this pause, which will be referred to as "hold" in the exercise instructions. Continue to breathe evenly and regularly.

After doing each exercise, take a brief rest. This relaxation period is an important component of muscle activity. It prevents stiffness and the build-up of fatigue.

All movements (unless otherwise stated) should be slow and gentle. Be alert for any sign of resistance or hint of pain in your body. Never attempt to force a movement.

Whenever possible, integrate imagery into the exercises to enhance their effectiveness. Try to visualize, for example, the release of tension; blood flowing unobstructed; a lessening of fatigue; feelings of warmth and comfort. Suggestions will be given from time to time with the exercise instructions.

GENERAL CAUTIONS

Before starting this or any other exercise regime or programme, you should always check with your doctor and obtain permission to do so.

If you suffer from an ear or eye disorder, such as a detached retina, omit any practice of inverted postures such as the half and full shoulderstand (see pp.98–9, 100–1) and the dog stretch (see p.36), which is part of the Sun salutations in Chapter Two. Avoid rapid abdominal breathing, as in the dynamic cleansing breath (see p.38) if you have epilepsy. Avoid inverted postures and rapid abdominal breathing if you have high blood pressure or heart disease.

Omit practice of the inverted postures during your menstrual period.

If you have a hernia, you should omit the cobra (see p.36), which is part of the Sun salutations in Chapter Two. Check with your doctor before practising the Sun salutations if you have varicose veins or venous blood clots.

Pregnant women who have a history of actual or threatened miscarriage are cautioned not to do the exercises in the first three or four months of pregnancy. If the pregnancy is progressing normally, try the warm-ups in Chapter Two, omitting the lying twist (see pp.26–7, the rock-and-roll (see p.31) and the Sun salutations (see pp.33–7). But first check with your doctor.

Some postures are not recommended during pregnancy. These include those done lying on the abdomen, as in the cobra (see p.36). Avoid lying flat on your back after the first trimester (three months), since this can restrict the blood and oxygen flow to mother and foetus, by putting pressure on the inferior vena cava (the principal vein draining the lower part of the body). Avoid squatting after the 34th week of pregnancy, until your baby's head is fully engaged.

CHAPTER TWO

Preparing for the day

The first few minutes after waking up can set the pace and tone for the rest of the day. Tumbling out of bed, stumbling to the bathroom, gulping a cup of coffee, and dashing out of the house will start you off on a frenetic note. Heavy traffic will ensure that you arrive at school or work feeling under pressure. This chapter will help you to start your day calmly.

Warm-up exercises help to reduce the bodily stiffness that often occurs after spending many hours in bed. They raise body temperature slightly, improve blood circulation, and wake you up gently. They also improve the flexibility and range of motion of the body's joints.

Even before you get out of bed, you can make the transition from being asleep to waking up smoother and less jarring to the nerves than bolting out of bed. On waking, lie still and turn your attention to your breathing. Make it progressively deeper. Do about five sets of wrist rotations (see p.25) and ankle rotations (see p.32). Stretch from head to feet while inhaling, and release the stretch while exhaling. Sit near the edge of your bed for a minute or so of quiet reflection.

The warm-ups in this chapter are ideal for people with busy lifestyles as they can be integrated into the most hectic of schedules to prevent a build-up of tension. When tension is allowed to accumulate, it often progresses to fatigue, aches, and, not infrequently, to pain, thus detracting from your quality of life and work. Suggestions for incorporating the warm-ups into your daily activities are given in the Notes and Suggestions that follow some of the descriptions of the exercises' benefits.

Do all the exercises slowly (unless otherwise instructed) and with awareness, synchronizing your movements with regular breathing through your nose. Do not hold your breath at any time.

Neck stretches

These stretches are wonderful for helping to keep the cervical (neck) part of the spine flexible and healthy. They also exercise the neck, an area of the body where tension tends to lodge.

NOTES AND SUGGESTIONS

Many of our daily activities, such as driving a car, sitting at a desk or computer, or reading, require a bending forward of the head and the body. This bending can lead to muscle strain, to which the neck is particularly vulnerable.

To prevent strain, which can and often does progress to aches or pain, it is prudent to take periodic breaks to do compensatory exercises such as the neck stretches. They require you to bring your head upright, crown uppermost, and to realign your neck with the rest of your spine. This counteracts the potential ill effects of constantly looking downward.

Remember to synchronize your head movements with slow, smooth breathing.

1. Sit or stand comfortably, with the crown of your head uppermost. Relax your shoulders, arms, and hands.
2. Slowly turn your head as far to the right as you comfortably can (01).
3. Slowly turn your head as far to the left as you comfortably can (02).
4. Turn your head to face forward.
5. Support the back of your neck with your hands and slowly and carefully tilt your head back to gently stretch the front of your neck (03).
6. Bring your head upright. Relax your hands and arms.
7. Slowly tilt your chin toward your chest to gently stretch out the back of your neck (04).
8. Bring your head upright.
9. Repeat the whole range of exercises (steps 2 to 8) several times in succession.
10. Rest. Breathe regularly.

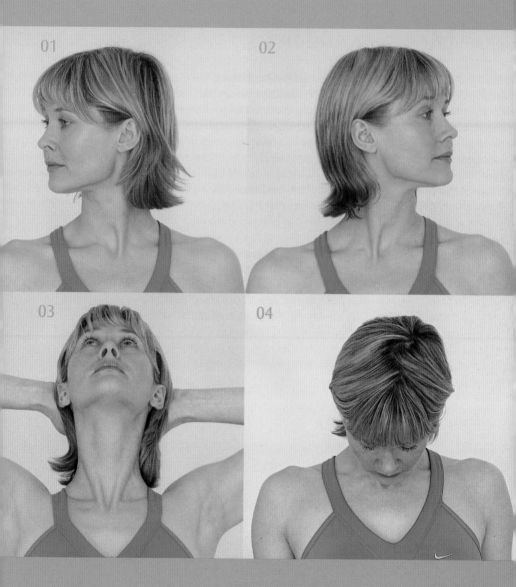

01

02

03

04

Ear-to-shoulder

The benefits of this warm-up are similar to those brought about by the neck stretches (see pp.18–19). It also exercises the platysma, a broad, flat layer of muscle that extends from each side of the neck to the jaw, so helping to maintain the contour of the neck and improving circulation to the face.

NOTES AND SUGGESTIONS
Practise the ear-to-shoulder whenever you can throughout the day, especially if you spend much of your time sitting at a desk or a computer, do a great deal of paperwork or reading, or engage in work that requires you to look down or bend forward frequently.

Practise the exercise during television advertising breaks, while waiting for the kettle to boil, or during tea and coffee breaks at your place of work. Look for opportunities to do this and other neck exercises. You may be surprised at how many there are, and you will be pleased to discover what relief such a seemingly simple exercise can bring.

1. Sit or stand comfortably. Keep your shoulders, arms, and hands relaxed. Relax your jaw and breathe regularly throughout the exercise.
2. Tilt your head sideways, aiming your right ear to your right shoulder (01).
3. Bring your head upright.
4. Tilt your head sideways, aiming your left ear to your left shoulder (02).
5. Bring your head upright.
6. Repeat the exercise (steps 2 to 5) several times.
7. Rest.

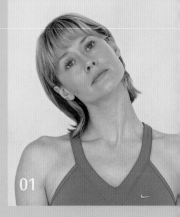

01

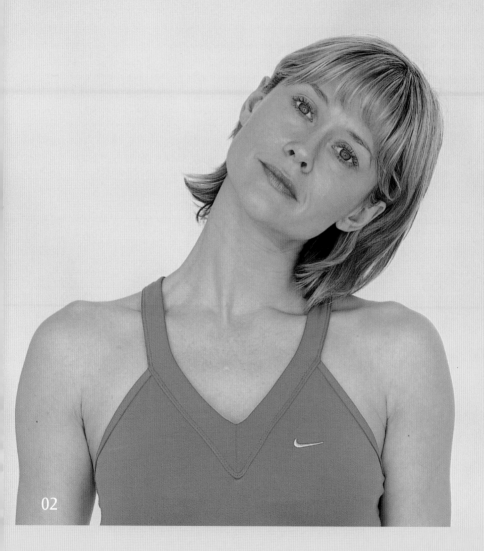

02

Shoulder shrugs

The shoulders and upper back are other favourite
areas for tension to lodge. Shoulder warm-ups
discourage tension build-up in the body and enhance
the effects of neck exercises. They counteract the
fatigue that often results from activities that require
much forward bending, and they contribute to
improved posture.

NOTES AND SUGGESTIONS
This simple exercise, practised frequently throughout
the day, will do much to prevent the tiredness and
tension that often result from spending many hours
at a desk, computer, or cash register, or, indeed,
from any job or activity that generates stress.

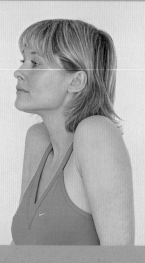

*1. Sit or stand comfortably
upright, with the crown of
your head uppermost. Relax
your arms and hands. Relax
your jaw and breathe regularly.
2. Pull your shoulders upward,
as if trying to touch your ears
with them (see left).
3. Hold the shrug for a few
seconds, but do not hold your
breath.
4. Relax your shoulders.
5. Repeat the exercise (steps 2
to 4) several times in succession.
6. Rest.*

Shoulder rotation

The benefits of this warm-up are the same as those produced by the shoulder shrugs (see p.22). In addition, shoulder rotation keeps the shoulder joints freely moving and so enhances range of motion and counteracts stiffness. It also conditions the accessory breathing muscles, which help the main respiratory (breathing) muscles during strenuous exercise and difficult breathing.

NOTES AND SUGGESTIONS

See the previous exercise (shoulder shrugs) for ideas on when to practise shoulder rotation.

When taking a warm shower, turn your back to the spray and practise shoulder rotation. It feels wonderful!

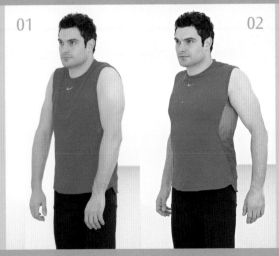

01   02

1. *Sit or stand comfortably upright, with the crown of your head uppermost. Relax your arms and hands. Then relax your jaw and breathe regularly.*
2. *Rotate your shoulders several times in a backward-forward direction (01–02).*
3. *Rest.*
4. *Repeat the exercise several times in a forward-backward direction.*
5. *Rest.*

Hands: the flower

Excellent for improving blood circulation in your hands, the flower also helps to keep your wrists and fingers supple. In addition, it prevents tension from building up to the point where it causes pressure on the nerves with resulting pain.

NOTES AND SUGGESTIONS

When you regularly do a great deal of typing or spend many hours working at a keyboard or cash register, the tendons that move your fingers can swell and exert pressure on the median nerve which runs through the wrist and controls much of the movement, feeling, and strength of the hand. This can result in soreness, tenderness, and weakness of the thumb muscles, and to numbness and weakness of the fingers or inability to bend them; it can also cause pain. Such symptoms are characteristic of a condition known as carpal tunnel syndrome (CTS), and if they persist you should consult your doctor.

1. Sit or stand comfortably upright, with the crown of your head uppermost. Relax your shoulders. Relax your jaw and breathe regularly.
2. Hold your hands, made into tight fists, in front of you (01).
3. Slowly, with resistance, open your hands (02).
4. Spread out your fingers, and stretch them fully.
5. As a follow-through, you may stretch your arms sideways and hold the stretch for a few seconds while continuing to breathe regularly.
6. Relax your arms and hands.
7. Finish the exercise by shaking your hands vigorously a few times, as if trying to rid them of water.
8. Rest.

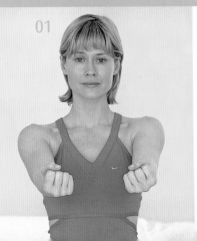

01

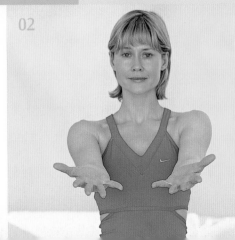

02

Wrist rotation

The benefits of regularly rotating your wrists are the same as those derived from practising the flower exercise (see p.24).

NOTES AND SUGGESTIONS
Look for opportunities throughout the day to do wrist rotation and other hand and finger exercises. You may do them, for example, during television advertising breaks or between chores.

I do six to eight wrist rotations in each direction before getting up in the morning. This simple procedure has kept my hands pain-free and fully functional over the many years that I have done a great deal of writing and typing.

1. Sit or stand comfortably upright. Relax your shoulders. Relax your jaw and breathe regularly.
2. Rotate your wrists several times in slow, smooth succession, as if drawing circles in the air with your hands: move your left hand clockwise and your right hand counterclockwise (01).
3. Rest your hands briefly.
4. Repeat the exercise (step 2) several times in the opposite direction (02).
5. You may complete the exercise by shaking your hands vigorously a few times, as though trying to rid them of water.

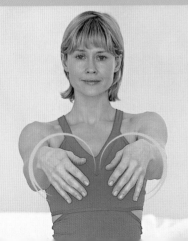

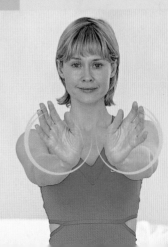

Lower back: the lying twist

This is an exercise in gentle torsion (twisting), which is necessary for a healthy back. It is also of benefit in toning the abdominal muscles, the condition of which affects the health of the spine.

NOTES AND SUGGESTIONS

The lower back (lumbar area), between the chest and the pelvis, is one of the structural weak points of the human spine. You can do much to ease back fatigue and to prevent backache by regularly doing strengthening and tension-relieving exercises such as the lying twist or its variation.

You may want to try doing it in bed (not a waterbed) before getting up in the morning, to counteract any stiffness that may have occurred overnight. Consider doing it on a carpeted floor when you come home from work, before doing your evening tasks, to remove residual kinks in your back after a day on your feet or sitting on a chair.

1. Lie on your back, with your arms sideways at shoulder level. Relax your jaw and breathe regularly.
2. Bend your legs, one at a time, and bring your knees toward your chest (01).
3. Keeping your shoulders and arms in firm contact with the surface on which you are lying, slowly, gently, and smoothly tilt your knees to one side as you exhale. You may keep your head still (02) or turn it to the side opposite the tilted knees.
4. Inhale and bring your knees to the centre.
5. Exhale and tilt your knees to the opposite side, keeping your head still or turning it to face opposite the tilted knees.
6. Repeat the side-to-side tilting of your knees (steps 3 to 5) several times in slow, smooth succession.
7. Bring your knees to the centre again (03). Stretch out your legs, one at a time. Relax your arms and hands.
8. Rest.

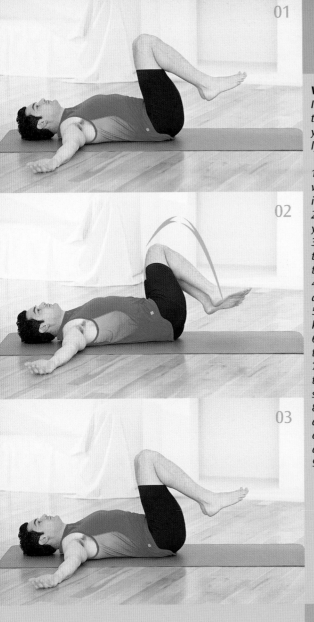

01

VARIATION
In the variation of the lying twist you prop yourself on your elbows rather than lying on your back.

1. Start in a sitting position, with your legs stretched out in front of you.
2. Lean back and prop yourself on your elbows.
3. Bend your legs, one at a time, and bring your knees toward your chest.
4. Tilt your knees to one side as you exhale.
5. Inhale and bring your knees to the centre.
6. Exhale and tilt your knees to the opposite side.
7. Repeat steps 4 to 6 several times in slow, smooth succession.
8. Bring your knees to the centre. Stretch out your legs, one at a time. Relax your arms and hands.
9. Rest.

02

03

Hips, legs, and thighs: the butterfly

The butterfly helps to reduce stiffness and promote flexibility in the ankle, knee, and hip joints. It gently stretches the adductor muscles which run along the inside of the thighs. It also improves circulation to the lower pelvis and the legs.

NOTES AND SUGGESTIONS
This is excellent for women's reproductive health.
You can do as many as 60 repetitions per minute while watching television or waiting for a kettle to boil.

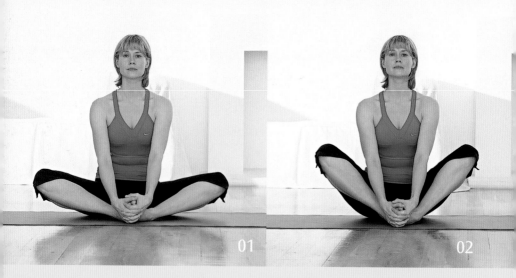

01   02

1. Sit upright with your legs folded inward, and the soles of your feet together. Clasp your hands around your feet and bring them comfortably close to your body (01).

2. Alternately lower your knees and raise them, like a butterfly flapping its wings (02). Do so as many times as you wish, at a slow to moderate pace.

3. Relax your arms and hands, and stretch out your legs, one at a time.

4. Rest.

VARIATION

1. Sit with your legs folded inward and the soles of your feet together. Pull your feet a comfortable distance from your body.

2. Support yourself by putting your hands flat on the mat beside you (03).

3. Alternately lower and raise your knees, as many times as you wish, at a slow to moderate pace (04).

4. Relax your arms and hands. Stretch out your legs, one at a time.

5. Rest.

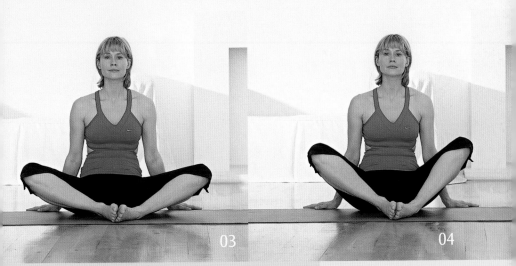

03

04

Spine and whole body: rock-and-roll

This is an excellent warm-up which conditions the
back and the abdominal muscles. It also exercises the
hamstring muscles at the back of the legs, which tend
to stiffen and shorten when you spend a lot of time
sitting. (The hamstrings affect the tilt of the pelvis, and
so have a bearing on posture, as well as on the health
of the back.)

   In addition, when you practise the rock-and-roll, you
press on 64 traditional acupressure points, with
general health benefits.

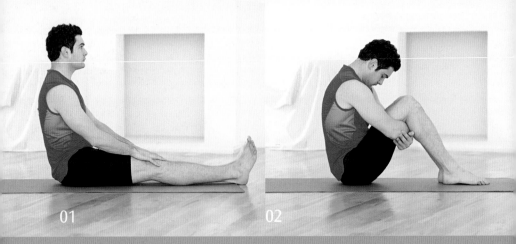

01

02

1. *Sit on a mat with your legs stretched out in front of you (01). Bend your legs and place the soles of your feet flat on the mat, close to your buttocks.*

2. *Pass your arms under your bent knees and hug your thighs. Tuck your head down and your chin in, making your back as rounded as you comfortably can (02). Relax your jaw and breathe regularly.*

3. *Inhale and kick your legs back to help you roll on to your back (03).*

4. *Exhale and rock forward into a sitting position again. Do not land heavily on your feet as the impact will jar your spine.*

5. *Repeat the rock-and-roll movements (steps 3 and 4), as many times as you wish, in smooth succession.*

6. *Sit or lie down and rest.*

NOTES AND SUGGESTIONS

The rock-and-roll is a good all-over morning warm-up to generate alertness and energy for the day's work. It takes only a minute or two to do between 10 and 20 repetitions. Choose a pace with which you feel completely comfortable.

Another superb all-body warm-up is the Sun salutation series which follows (see pp.33–7).

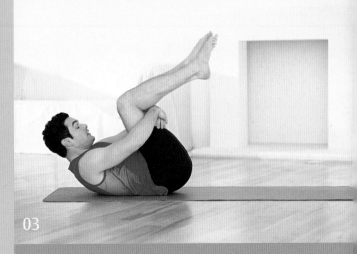

03

Ankles, feet, and legs: ankle rotation

Rotating your ankles is an excellent way of improving the circulation in your feet and legs, and increasing flexibility in the ankle joints.

NOTES AND SUGGESTIONS
Circulation in the feet and legs tends to slow down when we sit a great deal, and the feet may become cold. Rotating the ankles during periodic breaks is one way to help to maintain good circulation in the legs and feet. You can do this simple yet effective exercise in the office, at rest areas along the way during a long trip by car or bus, or while watching television. You can do it as soon as you wake up in the morning, while sitting near the edge of the bed, feet dangling.

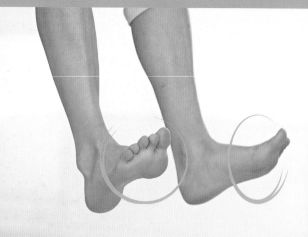

1. Sit where you can move your feet freely. Relax your jaw and breathe regularly throughout the exercise.
2. Make imaginary circles in the air with your feet: rotate the left ankle clockwise and the right ankle counterclockwise.
3. Repeat step 2 in the opposite direction, several times in slow, smooth succession: rotate the left ankle counterclockwise and the right ankle clockwise.
4. Relax your feet and legs.

The Sun salutations

Many of us spend several hours each day sitting at a desk, behind the wheel of a motor vehicle, or in front of a television set. Many others of us are on our feet for countless hours, either walking from place to place or standing at a counter, for example.

Such activities or inactivity put us at risk of becoming inflexible. Our joints stiffen from disuse and our muscles atrophy (waste away) to some extent from failure to receive normal exercise. An inflexible body is less efficient and more vulnerable to aches, pains, and injury than a flexible one. It is also unlikely to be as trim and energetic. Keeping flexible promotes fitness, energy, stamina, and resilience. It contributes to productivity and to the confidence that comes from feeling good about yourself.

The Sun salutations, consisting of 12 movements, promote the flexibility of the whole body. Each flows gracefully into the next, exercising the spine backward and forward, and stretching and toning the legs. They are done in synchronization with regular breathing and with total awareness.

Some of the movements, such as the cobra (step 7, p.36), can be practised as individual asanas (postures or exercises). Or the entire Sun salutation series can be used as the basis for a mini-workout of your own devising by adding a sideways-bending exercise and/or a spinal twist, so that all four sets of the muscles that form the "abdominal corset" and the complementary spinal muscles may be exercised during the same yoga practice session.

CAUTIONS
■ *If you have varicose veins or venous blood clots please check with your doctor before attempting to practise the Sun salutations.*
■ *Please also review the section on general cautions in Chapter One (see p.15).*

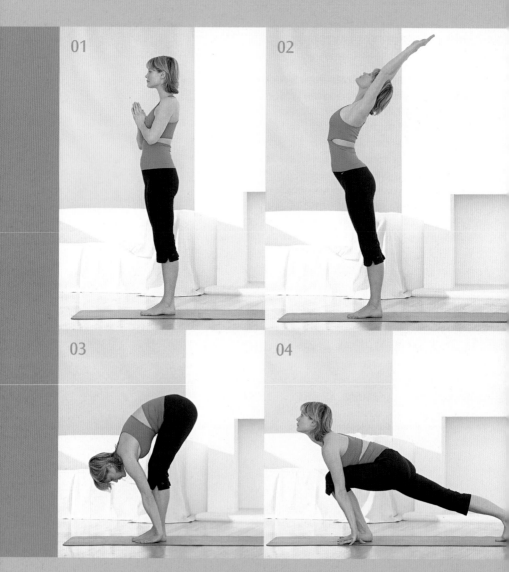

1. Stand tall, with the palms of your hands together in front of you as if in prayer (01). Relax your jaw and breathe regularly.
2. Inhale, stretch your arms overhead, and carefully bend backward. Tighten your buttock muscles to protect your back (02).
3. Exhale and bend forward, at your hip joints rather than at your waist, and place your hands on the mat beside your feet (03). Bend your knees, if necessary. As you gain flexibility, you will be able to keep your legs straight.
4. Inhale and look up. Taking the weight of your body on both hands, step back with your right foot, keeping your toes pointing firmly forward (04).
5. Neither inhaling nor exhaling, step back with your left foot. Your body weight is now borne by your hands and feet and is in a straight line from the back of your head to your heels (05).
6. Exhale and lower your knees to the mat. Also lower your chin (or forehead) and chest to the mat. This is the "knee-chest" or "eight points" position (06).

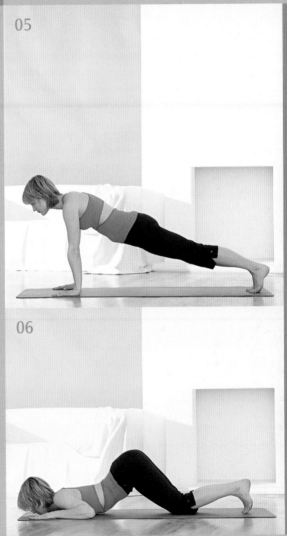

05

06

7. Inhaling, relax your feet so that your toes point backward. Lower your body to the mat and arch your back slowly and carefully. Keep your head up and your hands and hips in contact with the mat (07). This is the cobra posture.

8. Exhale and point your toes forward, pushing against the mat with your hands to help you raise your hips. Keep your arms as straight as you can and hang your head down. Aim your heels toward the mat but do not strain your hamstring muscles (08). This is the dog stretch posture.

9. Inhaling, look up, rock forward on to your toes, and step between your hands with your right foot (09).

10. Exhaling, step between your hands with your left foot and bend forward (10).

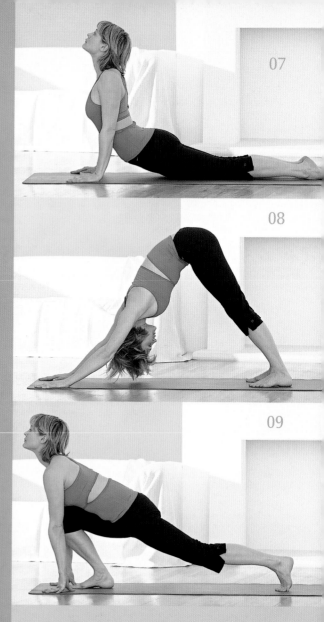

COOLING DOWN

After any exercise session it is important to cool down. This provides a chance for static muscle stretching, which enhances flexibility. It allows your cardio-vascular system (heart and blood vessels) to return gradually to normal functioning. It helps to prevent a sudden drop in blood pressure and, in addition, it permits metabolic waste products to be removed from the body, and energy reserves to be replenished.

All the exercises in this chapter, except the rock-and-roll, may be done as cooling-down exercises. Observe good posture when doing them and practise slowly. You may finish your session with a top-to-toe relaxation such as the pose of tranquillity described in Chapter Five (see pp.102–7).

11. Inhaling, come up carefully into a standing position, and move smoothly into a backward bend, with your arms overhead (11).
12. Exhale and resume your starting position (12).
Repeat all 12 movements, as many times as you wish, alternating the leading leg (see steps 4 and 9) each time.
13. Rest.

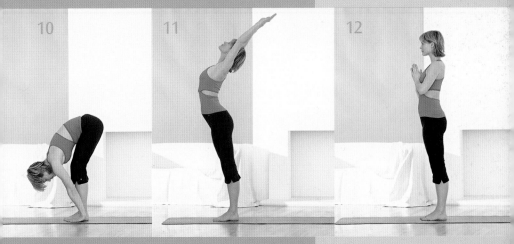

Dynamic cleansing breath

A good way in which to help yourself to wake up after a night's sleep is to practise this invigorating breathing exercise. It is also known as the "bellows' breath", the "runner's breath", and the "breath of fire", all of which give some indication of its powerful effects. It takes only about 30 seconds to do 30 of these respirations.

WHAT IT DOES

Wonderful for cleansing the sinuses and other respiratory passages, the dynamic cleansing breath also strengthens the diaphragm, a dome-shaped muscle that separates the chest and abdominal area. It gives a therapeutic massage to the abdominal organs and provides relief for those who suffer from breathing difficulties such as asthma.

The dynamic cleansing breath is also an excellent technique to practise whenever your energy levels drop too low.

CAUTIONS
- *Do not practise the dynamic cleansing breath if you suffer from any of the following: high blood pressure, epilepsy, hernia, an ear or eye disorder, or a herniated ("slipped") disc.*
- *Do not practise it during menstruation or pregnancy.*
- *Wait for at least two or three hours after eating to practise this exercise.*

NOTES AND SUGGESTIONS

You may practise the dynamic cleansing breath while lying down. The abdominal action and the sound of the breath when this exercise is performed are reminiscent of the expanding and collapsing of a bellows as it drives a blast of air into a fire. Visualizing this may help to grasp and master the technique.

Practise the exercise outdoors whenever you can, provided the air is relatively unpolluted.

The dynamic cleansing breath is completely different from hyperventilation (overbreathing): it is done consciously and purposefully, whereas hyperventilation is involuntary. The exercise results in thorough exhalation and, consequently, a full, spontaneous inhalation. In hyperventilation, carbon dioxide stores are quickly depleted, with unpleasant effects which include feelings of light-headedness and anxiety. This does not occur during the practice of the dynamic cleansing breath.

1. Sit or stand comfortably. Relax your shoulders, arms, and hands. Close your eyes or keep them open, as you prefer. Relax your jaw and breathe regularly.
2. Inhale slowly, smoothly, and as fully as you can without strain.
3. Exhale briskly through your nose as if sneezing; focus your attention on your abdomen, which will tighten and flatten.
4. Inhalation will follow naturally as you relax your abdomen and chest.
5. Repeat steps 3 and 4 in rapid succession. Try to do so about six times to start with. Gradually increase the number of repetitions as your stamina improves and you become more familiar with the technique.
6. Resume regular breathing.

Travel in balance and harmony

Travelling is an inescapable part of life today. It can range from a daily commute to and from the workplace, to short trips for shopping and business, to family travel for holidays and reunions. And for increasing numbers of people, travel involves plane journeys, some of which last many hours.

What used to be a relatively low-stress and essentially pleasant activity has now become, for many of us, one that is fraught with apprehension, anxiety, and frustration. Population growth, more money, and more accessible air travel are only some of the contributory factors. City streets are now more congested than ever, traffic during peak hours is painfully slow, and aircraft cabins are generally less spacious, with a recycled air supply. But this gloomy picture is not without relief, and you can do much to find this relief by using your own built-in resources of body, mind, and breath.

Apart from travel by public transport, driving to work is perhaps the most common method of transport. It is also one of the most stressful. Before installing yourself behind the wheel in the morning, be sure to have an adequate breakfast as this will contribute to the alertness and evenness of temper you will need to cope with slow-moving traffic or with the lack of consideration shown by some of your fellow motorists.

Four breathing techniques that you can practise en route are described in this chapter. Key points to remember when doing them are: maintaining good posture, with the crown of your head uppermost; relaxing your body as much as you can, paying particular attention to your lips, jaw, and tongue; breathing in and out through your nose (unless instructed otherwise), and keeping your breathing rhythm slow and even.

Anti-anxiety breath

Although the link between respiration and physical states may be readily apparent, the connection between breathing and mental states, while perhaps not immediately obvious, is nevertheless undeniable. Changes in feelings, particularly if they are intense, are reflected in patterns of breathing and can profoundly affect the smooth, continuous flow of breath. But since the relationship between breath and mind is reciprocal, you can bring about a change in emotional climate by consciously altering your breathing pattern.

WHAT IT DOES

This is an excellent exercise to practise before you drive and whenever you are apprehensive or worried; when you are facing a challenging or dreaded situation; when you are tempted to act impulsively. It will help you to maintain control over your actions.

1. Check your posture: make sure that your head is naturally poised, your chin neither too far down nor up. Do not clutch your steering-wheel like a weapon. Hold it securely but in a relaxed manner. Make sure that your seat is adjusted so that your legs can reach the pedals without being locked straight. Relax your knees. Sit as far back in your seat as you comfortably can. Relax your shoulders and your jaw and breathe regularly.

2. Inhale quietly through your nose, slowly, smoothly, and as completely as you can without force.

3. Exhale through your nose slowly, smoothly, and as thoroughly as you can without strain.

4. Before inhaling again mentally count: "One thousand, two thousand". This will prevent you hyperventilating.

5. Repeat steps 2 to 4 in smooth succession, until your breathing rate has become slower and you feel calmer.

6. Resume regular breathing.

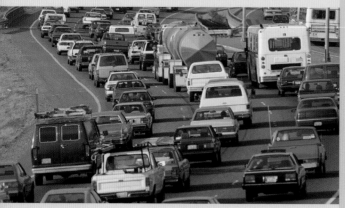

Sighing breath

This is a wonderful technique for releasing pent-up emotion and for managing stress. Practise it whenever you sense tension mounting or whenever you feel anxious or frustrated.

NOTES AND SUGGESTIONS
The sighing breath is also known as "pursed-lip breathing". It helps to prolong your exhalation and so promotes a sense of control over your respiration, a process that is both involuntary and voluntary. It is useful in combating difficult breathing (dyspnoea) and the sense of panic that can accompany it.

Do not feel self-conscious about practising this exercise while sitting in a tailback or a layby. People will think you are whistling.

1. Check your posture (see step 1 of the anti-anxiety breath, p.42). Relax your jaw and breathe regularly.
2. Inhale slowly, smoothly, and as deeply as you comfortably can through your nostrils.
3. Exhale steadily through pouted lips, as if whistling or cooling a hot drink (see below left). Close your mouth at the end of the exhalation, but do not tighten your jaw or compress your lips.
4. Repeat steps 2 and 3 in smooth succession, as many times as you wish.
5. Resume regular breathing.

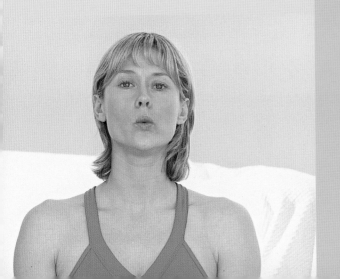

Sniffing breath

When your chest is so tight that you are unable to take a comfortably deep inward breath, the sniffing breath is the exercise that you should do. It is a wonderful antidote to the build-up of tension in the chest and elsewhere in the body.

NOTES AND SUGGESTIONS
Practising the sniffing breath whenever you feel anxious, upset, or under pressure, will help you stay relaxed and in control.

1. Establish and maintain good posture. Relax your jaw and breathe regularly.
2. Take two, three, or more small, quick inward breaths, as if you were breaking up your inhalation into small equal parts.
3. Exhale steadily through your nose or through pursed lips (see below).
4. Repeat steps 2 and 3 again, until you feel your chest relaxing and you can take one deep inward breath without straining.
5. Resume regular breathing.

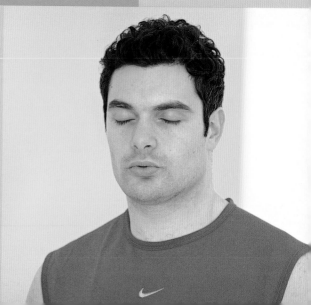

Ujjayi pranayama

The Sanskrit word ujjayi means "control or victory through expansion". Pranayama is the word used to describe yoga's breathing exercises. Ujjayi pranayama is sometimes referred to as "breath with sound" or "the victorious breath".

WHAT IT DOES
This breathing exercise improves the ventilation of the lungs, calms frayed nerves, and replenishes energy. It helps to slow down the heartbeat and so ease the heart's workload. It also contributes to a strengthening of the immune system, which protects the body from invasion by harmful organisms.

As an introduction to this technique, imagine that you're blowing on to a windowpane to make it foggy by whispering the syllable "haa" (see below left). This will help you to bring about the relaxation of your throat that is necessary for the correct execution of the breathing exercise itself. Now you're ready to begin.
1. Relax your jaw, keeping your lips closed though not compressed. Inhale slowly through your nose while pretending to say "haa".
2. Exhale slowly and completely through your nose, with your mouth still closed, while again pretending to say "haa".
3. Repeat steps 1 and 2 again and again in smooth succession. Listen for a smooth, even sound, which will indicate calm, in contrast with a rough, uneven one, which suggests some agitation.
4. Resume regular breathing.

Longer road journeys

The demands of a long journey by road can tax the driver's resources to the limit and put a strain on the interpersonal relationships of the vehicle's occupants. The key to avoiding this is to forestall the build-up of tension which can be insidious. By practising simple exercises en route and also at rest stops along the way, there is a good chance that you can expect to arrive at your destination with energy to spare, rather than exhausted and bad-tempered.

When you arrive at your destination, you will benefit from taking a few moments to rest your eyes and, indeed, your whole body and your mind. Sit somewhere comfortable or lie down, close your eyes, and practise any of the breathing exercises described in this chapter. For a top-to-toe relaxation that is perhaps without match, practise the pose of tranquillity, described in Chapter Five (see pp.102–7; see also below).

EVERY LITTLE HELPS
Although the exercises you will be incorporating each day into your activities are simple and take very little time, do not think that they are insignificant. Their effects are cumulative; what really counts is the regularity with which you integrate them into your daily life.

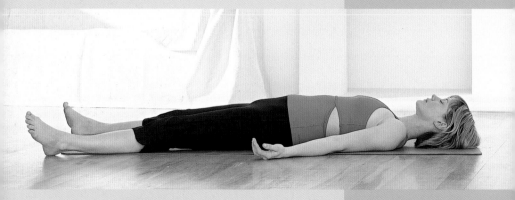

Eyes: palming

Drivers expend a great deal of energy through their
eyes. After hours of defensive driving, the eyes can
become very strained. Park your vehicle safely and
practise the following exercise to counteract eye strain,
prevent tension build-up in your face and body, and
promote concentration.

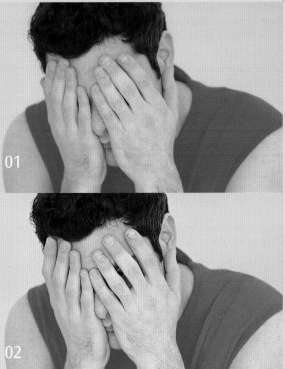

*1. Sit where you can rest your
elbows: on a picnic table or
even on the steering-wheel of
your parked car.*
*2. Rub your palms together
vigorously to warm them up.*
*3. Rest your palms gently over
your closed eyes to shut out
the light. Do not put pressure
on your eyeballs (01). Relax
your jaw. Breathe regularly.*
*4. Stay in this position for a
minute or two. If you wish,
you may keep your eyes closed
but again rub your palms
together and continue the
palming for a further minute
or two.*
*5. Separate your fingers so
that the light is slowly
reintroduced (02). Relax your
arms and hands.*
*6. To finish the exercise, blink
several times to lubricate your
eyes with natural moisture.*

Neck, shoulders, and limbs

THE NECK
With your vehicle safely parked, sit on a log, bench, or boulder, and with your eyes either closed or open, practise neck stretches (see pp.18–19) (01, 02) and the ear-to-shoulder exercise (see pp.20–1).

THE SHOULDERS
Sit on a suitable prop, such as a bench or a fallen tree, or even on the grass. You may also stand. Relax your jaw and breathe regularly. Shrug your shoulders (see p.22) and do shoulder rotations (see p.23).

You may also try one or both of the exercises for the shoulders and upper back: the chest expander (see p.58) and the posture clasp (see p.59), which have the added benefit of improving posture.

ARMS AND HANDS
While sitting or standing, practise the flower (see p.24) (03, 04) and wrist rotation (see p.25).

FEET AND LEGS
Find a prop on which you can sit and freely move your legs. Practise ankle rotation (see p.32). You may also alternately bend and straighten your legs to keep the knee joints moving freely and improve circulation.

HIDDEN RESOURCES
Let us not forget the rich, largely untapped store of personal resources we have within us wherever we are: our powers of concentration, our ability to form mental pictures, and our breath. Though they are intangible and cost no money, these have the power to transform our lives. With faithful practice, we can become skilled in using these "tools" to improve our health, our productivity, and, indeed, our joy in living.

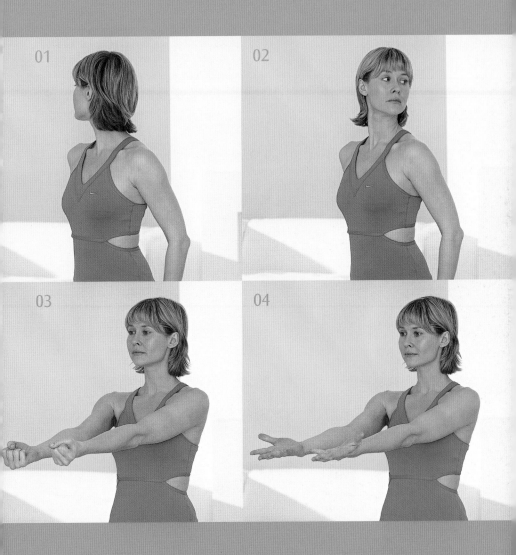

All-over stretching: the rag doll

Like any all-over stretch, synchronized with regular breathing, the rag doll will help to counteract bodily stiffness and replenish energy reserves.

NOTES AND SUGGESTIONS

Combine imagery with this exercise to enhance its relaxing effects. While dangling, visualize all your accumulated tiredness draining away.

You may also do the backward and forward bends in the Sun salutation series (see pp.34–5), and for a lateral (sideways) stretch you could include the half moon posture (see p.116).

1. Stand tall. Relax your arms at your sides. Relax your jaw and breathe regularly.
2. Tilt your head forward, bringing your chin toward your chest.
3. Let your shoulders droop and keep your arms and hands limp.
4. Slowly curl your body forward. Let the weight of your arms pull your body down until it hangs loosely. Dangle your arms (see left).
5. Stay in this posture for as long as you wish while breathing regularly.
6. Slowly uncurl your body until you are once again standing upright.
7. Sit or lie down and rest.

CAUTION
■ *The rag doll may not be appropriate if you have a history of high blood pressure. Please check with your doctor.*

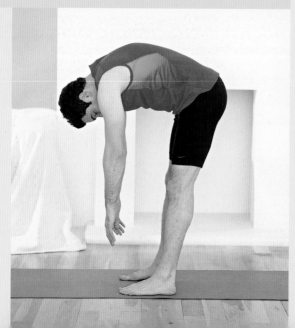

Air travel

Whereas road travel offers opportunities to park at convenient areas along the way to practise certain tension-relieving exercises, air travel does not. Nevertheless, there are many in-flight techniques that you can use to reduce the stress of flying and help to make it a pleasant experience.

AT THE AIRPORT

With the phenomenal increase in air travel in recent years, there has been a higher incidence of flight delays. Waiting at airports can be tedious, and there is only so much reading you can do while waiting to board the plane, before both your eyes and your whole body begin to feel fatigued.

Since you may not wish to practise exercises that call attention to yourself, why not use a tool that you carry with you everywhere, your breath? Practise the anti-anxiety breath (see p.42) and the sniffing breath (see p.44), both of which can be done unobtrusively. Or you may wish to try a simple breath meditation, known as breath observation (see p.52), which will divert your attention from the delay and its concomitant frustration, and will reduce tension build-up, promoting a sense of calm and control.

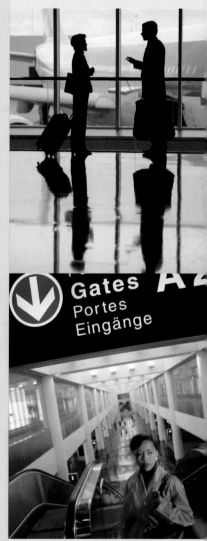

Breath observation

The object of this exercise is to keep your attention on the breathing cycle and to contemplate it. Start with a couple of minutes of practice, and increase the time as you become more familiar and comfortable with it.

NOTES AND SUGGESTIONS
Once in the cabin you may practise any of the breathing exercises referred to in the previous section. Remember to relax your jaw by unclenching your teeth. This has the added advantage of discouraging the facial tension that can lead to headaches.

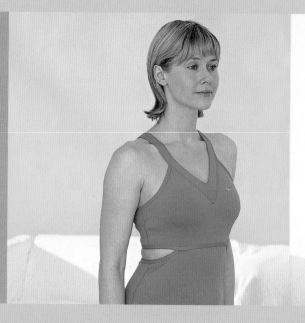

1. Sit or stand comfortably, with good posture. Relax your shoulders and hands. Relax your jaw and breathe regularly (see right).
2. With your eyes open or closed, focus your attention only on your breathing, without manipulating it in any way. Become a silent observer of your own breathing process: note the rate of breathing, the depth or shallowness, the smoothness or unevenness, the sounds of quietness, and the natural pause that occurs between exhalation and inhalation.

Shoulders, back, legs, and feet

SHOULDERS AND UPPER BACK
To prevent an accumulation of tension in your
shoulders and upper back, squeeze your shoulder
blades together while inhaling and relax them while
exhaling. Do this a few times in succession. No one
will know what you are doing.

LOWER BACK
Keep the small of your back (waist level) well
supported with a small cushion or a rolled-up garment
or towel. Practise pelvic tilting, as follows (see also
pp.60–1), to discourage backache and back fatigue.
Inhale slowly and smoothly through your nose.

As you exhale steadily, press the small of your back
toward the back of your chair.

Hold the pressure as long as your exhalation lasts.
Inhale and relax your back. Repeat several times.
Relax, breathing regularly.

LEGS AND FEET
Unless you are travelling in a cabin with ample space
to stretch out your legs, it may be difficult to do
exercises to maintain good circulation in the legs and
feet, but you can practise ankle rotation (see p.32).
On a long flight, you can periodically walk to the
washroom, where you can also take the opportunity
of doing a few neck stretches (see pp.18–19) and ear-
to-shoulder exercises (see pp.20–1).

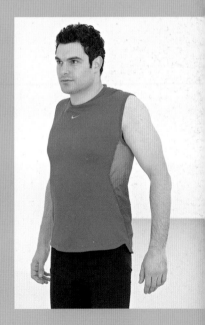

CHAPTER FOUR

Yoga at work

With the exception of the self-employed, the workplace, for many of us, has become a fast-paced, high-pressure environment. Each day we are confronted with such challenges as deadlines, uncertainty about job security, and various frustrations that include those connected with our interpersonal relationships. Is it any wonder, then, that we often return home feeling exhausted, drained, and discouraged?

The number of hours we spend at our place of work each year represents a significant portion of our lives. What a waste it is if work is seen as a necessary evil rather than something satisfying and meaningful. Even if you're not among the remarkably lucky few who love what they do so passionately that they cannot differentiate it from being on vacation, there are simple, effective measures you can take to counteract the stresses inherent in the work environment. You can practise yoga at work. You can practise it, too, even if you have a home-based business.

Before looking for outside solutions to difficulties that arise from time to time, start first with something you have with you wherever you are: your breath. It is perhaps your most underutilized stress reduction "tool". Try this: when next you feel anxious, angry, or frightened, unclench your teeth, keeping your lips together but not compressed. Slow down your rate of breathing. Breathe in and out through your nose but pretend you are breathing through your mouth. You'll be amazed at how quickly this will relax your chest and allow you to breathe more deeply and easily. And because breathing and emotions are very closely linked, you will experience a noticeable lessening of your anxiety, anger, or fear.

At the same time, relax your hands instead of making them into fists. Form a mental picture in which you see your tension escaping through your hands. Check your facial muscles also, replacing a frown with a smile.

Eyes

Many of us spend hours each day working at a computer, reading, writing, or doing other close work. With the possible addition of glare, our eyes become very vulnerable to eye strain, which can contribute to headaches or a general feeling of fatigue.

Take a short break about once every hour and practise one or two of the following eye exercises, some of which may even be done at your desk.

NOTES AND SUGGESTIONS

Glare is considered the single biggest cause of eye strain, especially when you use a computer. Here are some suggestions for protecting your eyes.

Avoid placing your monitor in direct light, sunlight, or other light source.

Fluorescent overhead lights are notorious for causing glare. Consider turning off those directly above your monitor, and perhaps using a small portable light instead.

Consider also the use of a glare screen, available at computer stores, which can be attached to the front of your monitor.

Check with your eye specialist about using spectacles for glare prevention, even if you don't need a prescription to correct your sight.

Avoid staring at the screen for long periods without a break. This tends to produce dryness of the eyes. Periodically, look at a distant object and blink several times, as described in the first two eye exercises.

1. Look away from your monitor or other work source. Focus your attention for several seconds, or a minute or more, on a distant object, while checking that you are breathing regularly with your teeth unclenched and your jaw relaxed.

2. Blink your eyes frequently to moisturize them with natural fluid.

3. Put your eye muscles through a range of motion to strengthen and also relax them. With your head still, the crown uppermost, and your shoulders relaxed, look to your left, then to your right. Look up, then down. Repeat these four movements several times. Keep your jaw relaxed.

4. Practise palming (see p.47) to give your eyes relief from light and glare.

Neck, shoulders, and upper back

THE NECK

Neck pain is frequently reported to doctors. Among its causes are prolonged sitting on chairs or at the wheel of vehicles, poor posture, and an unrelieved bending forward of the head. This results in muscle strain and pressure on nerves, which can also contribute to headaches.

To compensate for constantly looking downward, to prevent a build-up of tension, fatigue, and pain in the neck and adjacent areas, and to maintain feelings of comfort, take short periodic breaks from work and practise the neck stretches (see pp.18–19) and the ear-to-shoulder exercises (see pp.20–1).

If it is not convenient to do these exercises at your desk, look for a place where you can practise them inconspicuously, such as in a washroom, behind a filing cabinet, or even in your car while parked.

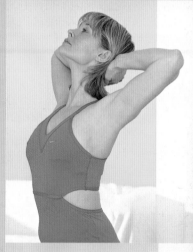

THE SHOULDERS AND UPPER BACK

Two favourite areas for tension to lodge and accumulate are the shoulders and upper back. Activities requiring a lot of bending forward tend to promote this, as does habitual poor posture.

To decrease the incidence of problems related to tension build-up and strain in the shoulders and upper back, practise shoulder shrugs (see p.22) and shoulder rotation (see p.23) during short breaks from work. You could also try the chest expander (see p.58) and the posture clasp (see p.59) whenever you can.

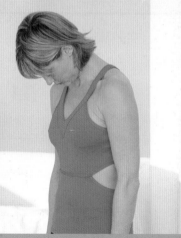

Chest expander

This exercise is superb for reducing tension build-up in your shoulders and upper back. It also helps to improve posture and facilitates deep breathing.

NOTES AND SUGGESTIONS
Practise the chest expander throughout your work day if you spend a great deal of time at a desk or engaged in activities that require you to bend forward.

1. *Stand tall, with the crown of your head uppermost and your arms relaxed at your sides. You may also practise this exercise sitting where you can swing your arms freely behind you. Relax your jaw and breathe regularly.*
2. *Swing your arms behind you and interlace the fingers of one hand with those of the other. Stay upright.*
3. *Raise your arms upward to their comfortable limit and keep them straight (see left).*
4. *Hold the raised-arms posture as long as you comfortably can while breathing regularly.*
5. *Lower and relax your arms and hands.*
6. *You may finish by shrugging or rotating your shoulders a few times.*
7. *Rest.*

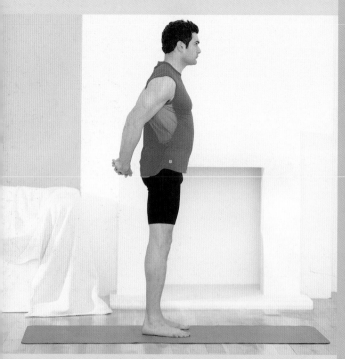

Posture clasp

The posture clasp helps to prevent stiffness in the arm and shoulder joints, keeping them freely moving. It also counteracts the effects of poor postural habits.

NOTES AND SUGGESTIONS
If you can't interlock your fingers in step 3, use a scarf to extend your arms: toss one end over your shoulder, reaching behind and below to grasp the other end.

1. *Sit or stand tall, with the crown of your head uppermost. Relax your jaw and breathe regularly.*
2. *Reach over your right shoulder with your right hand. Point your elbow upward rather than forward, and keep your arm close to your ear (01).*
3. *With your left hand, reach behind your back, from below, and interlock your fingers with those of your right hand (02).*
4. *Hold this posture as long as you comfortably can while breathing regularly.*
5. *Resume your starting position and rest briefly.*
6. *Repeat the exercise, changing arms, so that your left elbow now points upward (steps 2 to 5).*
7. *You may finish the exercise by shrugging your shoulders or rotating them a few times.*
8. *Rest.*

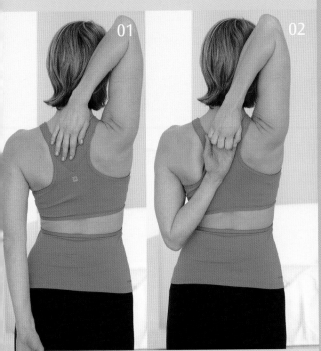

Lower back: standing and sitting pelvic tilt

Lower back pain is widespread but you can greatly decrease your chances of being a sufferer by incorporating a few simple measures into your daily activities. The pelvic tilt will help you to keep your back correctly aligned, thus reducing the likelihood of developing lower back pain.

NOTES AND SUGGESTIONS

Practise the sitting pelvic tilt at your desk, during meetings, in the cafeteria, or in your parked car.

Women can use both the sitting and standing version as ante- and postnatal exercises for strengthening the back and the abdomen.

Practise the standing version of the pelvic tilt several times throughout the day wherever you find a handy prop and can do it unobtrusively. You can try it while in a queue or even during a conversation, if you feel comfortable doing so.

STANDING VARIATION:

1. Find a suitable prop such as a post, the wall of an elevator, or a stable piece of furniture.
2. Stand with your back to your chosen prop and inhale slowly and smoothly through your nose.
3. Exhale and press the small of your back toward the prop. Hold the pressure for the duration of your exhalation (01).
4. Inhale. Relax your back (02).
5. Repeat steps 2 to 4 a few more times.
6. Rest.

SITTING VARIATION:

1. Inhale slowly and smoothly through your nose.
2. On your exhalation, press the small of your back (waist) toward the back of your chair.
3. Hold the pressure as long as your exhalation lasts.
4. Inhale. Relax your back.
5. Repeat steps 2 to 4 a few more times.
6. Rest.

01
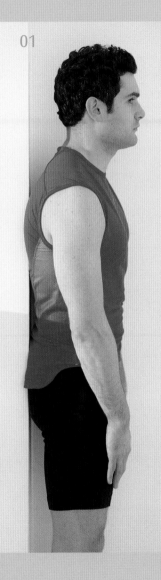

02
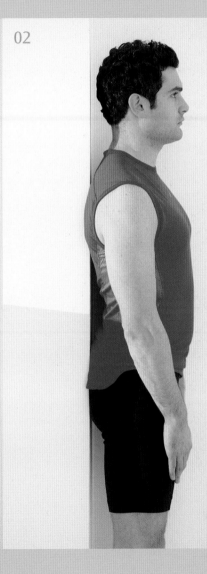

Hands and arms

Review the section on hands in Chapter Two. Take
frequent short breaks from your work and practise
the flower (see p.24) and wrist rotation (see p.25).
   Because the muscles of your wrists are connected
to those of your arms, shoulders, and neck, remember
to do appropriate exercises for those parts also.
The chest expander (see p.58) will give a therapeutic
stretch to your arms, and is a good complement to
the hand and wrist exercises.

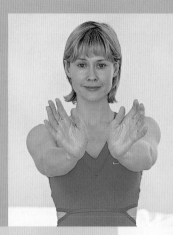

Legs and feet

Stretch out your legs periodically to help maintain
good circulation. Whenever you conveniently can,
practise ankle rotation (see p.32).
   Do not cross your legs while working, as it can
constrict blood flow and impair sensation, causing
your legs to tingle or "go to sleep".
   Find opportunities to walk: take the stairs instead of
the elevator. Take short walks outdoors, if facilities for
this are available, to stretch your leg muscles and give
a boost to your circulation. Do breathing exercises of
your choice while walking.

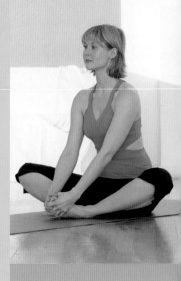

The whole body

Treat yourself during breaks throughout the day to a therapeutic all-over stretch: inhale and reach upward with both arms; exhale and lower and relax your arms. If you wish to stretch sideways, try the half moon (see p.116) or an appropriate modification. Finish with the rag doll (see p.50).

When I worked in hospital, I would often use my lunch break to replenish my reserves away from the hustle and bustle of the ward. After a customary bowl of soup and some wholegrain bread, I would go to a quiet spot on the grounds among the trees and flowers and sit in contemplation. Or I would retreat to the small Japanese-style garden surrounded by a bamboo fence and listen to the water trickling over the rocks or admire the foliage or the stone lanterns. Sometimes I would do a simple meditation. I would return to work feeling more tranquil than when I left, and a worthier resource for those who depended on me. This was in marked contrast with those times when I chose to remain in the cafeteria where the incessant chatter was not at all conducive to calm and composure.

On night shift, during my main break from work, I often did a lying version of an all-body stretch known as the stick posture, which can also be done while standing. It is a sustained top-to-toe stretch done while lying on the back, with the toes pulled toward the body and the arms overhead.

When the stretch was released, I would sink further into the surface on which I was lying with each exhalation. Within ten minutes, I would sense a noticeable lessening of my initial tension and fatigue.

Breath counting

Borrowed from the Zen masters, this apparently simple breathing exercise is extremely effective at calming the body and mind. It temporarily diverts your attention from everyday concerns and disturbing stimuli, and helps you to become more focused and consequently more in control of yourself and your life.

NOTES AND SUGGESTIONS
Do not count higher than four. If you find yourself at seven or eight or higher, you will know that your attention has strayed, and you will need to redirect it and start again at one.

Give your complete attention to the counting, synchronized with your breathing. When you are aware that your thoughts have strayed to other matters, gently but firmly bring them back to the counting and the breathing.

Finish your meditation gradually; you should never end abruptly.

1. Sit upright, with the crown of your head uppermost. Close your eyes or keep them open, as you prefer. Relax your jaw and breathe regularly. Let your breath come in and go out naturally, and as you progressively relax, it will become slower and smoother.
2. As you exhale, mentally count "one".
3. Inhale.
4. On the following exhalation, mentally count "two".
5. Repeat steps 2 and 3 in slow, smooth succession, up to a mental count of four.
6. Repeat steps 2 to 5, as often as you wish.
7. Resume regular breathing without counting.

Stress reduction

All the exercises in this book encourage self-observation and a heeding of your body's signals. This helps you to develop a sort of "tuning in" which will alert you to rising stress levels. You can then promptly take appropriate steps to prevent these levels from rising beyond your control.

Here are some tips you can apply at work and elsewhere to help you to cope with everyday stresses:

BE INFORMED
The more informed you are about stress, its signs and symptoms, and what it can do to you, the better equipped you will be to cope with it.

KEEP FIT
Attaining and maintaining the best possible level of fitness will give you stamina and resilience for dealing effectively with any difficulties that you encounter. All the asanas (postures or exercises) and breathing, relaxation, and meditation exercises in this book, practised regularly, will do much to promote optimum wellness. Incorporating the tension-relieving techniques into daily schedules will help to prevent the build-up of tension that may sometimes cause you to act impulsively, and which also generates fatigue, aches, and pains.

EMOTIONAL SUPPORT
It is vital that you establish and preserve a reliable emotional support system consisting of one or more people. This could be a trusted, dependable friend or friends; a professional counsellor with whom you have a good rapport; or a pastor or other spiritual advisor.

SOLID SUPPORT
A solid support system will provide you with inspiration when you feel discouraged, and a healthy outlet for feelings that are better expressed than suppressed. It will, moreover, reinforce positive emotions and promote a sense of self-worth and self-confidence, attributes that are often eroded when you feel dejected and hopeless.

ANGER MANAGEMENT

Learn to channel your anger into constructive outlets, such as exercise. Learn to speak up if you have a problem; to be assertive rather than aggressive. Make enquiries about anger management courses.

SMILE

During the first few seconds of a stressful situation try this: Smile inwardly and with your eyes and mouth. Take a slow, smooth inward breath, as deep as you can without straining. Exhale steadily while letting go of tightness in your jaw, tongue, hands, and shoulders. Tell yourself that you are calm, alert, and in control.

SIMPLIFY YOUR LIFE

Determine who and what are truly of most value to you and give most of your time and energy to those people and things. Resist the temptation to equate simplicity with deprivation.

SAY NO!

Learn to say "no". This is one of the most difficult stress-reduction strategies for many people to put into practice because of the associated feelings of guilt. The ability to say "no" firmly but graciously prevents the over-commitment that adds to the frustrations of a busy schedule.

PLAY FOR PLEASURE

Experts in the field of mental health agree that play is very important for well-being, which contributes to the ability to cope. Balance your work with a hobby or sport that you are passionate about or greatly enjoy. Avoid bringing a spirit of competition to your recreation.

SELF-ESTEEM

Love and respect yourself. Low self-esteem is a form of self-rejection, which is perhaps the ultimate stressor.

TIME MANAGEMENT

Effective time management is an essential part of stress reduction. But finding enough time for all the things you want or need to do can indeed be very stressful. It can result in a feeling of intense pressure, which sometimes borders on desperation. Once you learn to identify your priorities, devise a plan, and put it into action, you can relieve much of the distress. The key is to "work smart", rather than longer or harder.

Here are some tips to help you to avoid time- wasting:

Reduce Clutter
Clutter detracts from effectiveness. Keep your work areas and surroundings organized.

Use Your Time Wisely
Use part of your tea and coffee breaks to reduce tension build-up and replenish energy stores.

If you cannot reduce the time you spend commuting to and from work or driving children to and from various activities, then profit from travel time. You could listen to an educational cassette while driving, or share the school run with a friend.

Plan Your Work
Time spent planning is well invested as it saves time in the long run. It can avoid having to re-do a project.

Be Focused
Regularly practise some form of meditation to train you to be more centred and therefore to concentrate better. Explore your tendency to delay doing certain tasks – perhaps the most difficult ones –and try to find ways of overcoming this bad habit.

Protect yourself from interruptions. It is the amount of uninterrupted time devoted to a job that is significant.

Avoid Perfectionism
Perfectionism generates frustration, a powerful stressor. Strive instead for excellence of effort and performance.

Work Intelligently
Distinguish between those activities that bring positive results and those that merely pass the time.

Delegate Chores
Keep your home clean and reasonably tidy but not sterile. Delegate chores to family members.

Stay Well and Relax
Failure to take care of your health can result in days off work, which is another major time-waster. Nurture your spirit as well as your body: visit an art gallery, go to a concert, or go on a retreat. You will return to your normal activities with renewed enthusiasm, greater productivity, and an enhanced sense of accomplishment.

CHAPTER FIVE

Rest and relaxation

Home is a safe haven which offers us shelter and protection from the myriad stresses of the outside world. But that does not mean that it is without other challenges. When you get home from work you may well have chores to do, children to attend to, and meals to prepare. Nevertheless, home presents many opportunities for rest and relaxation.

On arriving home, try to reserve the first five or ten minutes to help you to adjust from the activities of the workplace and the hum of traffic. This is time very well spent as it can set the tone for the rest of the evening.

You can incorporate a number of yoga techniques into your evening agenda. While waiting for a kettle to boil or a meal to cook, for example, you could do a balancing posture to help strengthen your powers of concentration.

Other exercises you can do while working in the kitchen in the evening include the chest expander (see p.58) and the posture clasp (see p.59), which are two of my favourites. You can also practise most of the exercises described in Chapter Two, and you can benefit from the eye exercises in Chapter Four (see p.56). You may also want to try the meditation in action exercise (see p.82), which you can modify to suit you.

A good time to meditate is before you've eaten your evening meal. The firm posture (see p.85) and the easy pose (see pp.86–7) are ideal for meditation.

You can also practise breathing techniques while doing your chores. This is one of the quickest and most effective ways of combating fatigue, restoring energy, and promoting calm. First, do a quick mental head-to-toe check: release any tension in your jaw, lips, shoulders, and hands. Next, check your rate of breathing. If it's too fast, slow it down. If it's too shallow, do the sniffing breath (see p.44) and the sighing breath (see p.43).

Legs and feet: legs-up

The legs-up posture is wonderful for relieving tired, aching legs and feet. By helping the flow of blood from the legs to the heart, and lessening the wear and tear on the valves, it is also excellent for discouraging the formation of varicose veins.

NOTES AND SUGGESTIONS
Practise a breathing exercise of your choice or all-body breathing (see p.71) while in this posture.

CAUTION
Do not practise this posture if you have recently-formed blood clots.

1. *Lie facing a wall. Lift your legs and rest your feet against the wall, so that they form an angle of about 45 degrees with the surface on which you are lying (see below). You may also rest your feet on a sofa or other suitable prop.*
2. *Relax your arms, close your eyes, and breathe regularly. Stay here for as long as you can (five or ten minutes will suffice).*
3. *When you are ready, get up slowly and carefully: bring your knees toward your abdomen, roll on to your side, and come into a sitting position.*

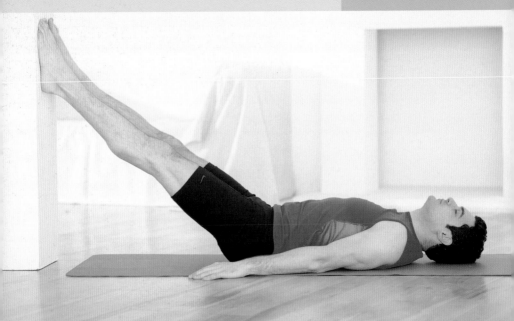

All-body breathing

All-body breathing enhances the ability to form pictures in your mind, known as visualization or imagery. It is not merely wishful thinking, daydreaming, or fantasizing, which are passive and unfocused. Visualization is active and purposeful.

During the past decade or two, researchers have discovered and documented that almost anyone can learn to control functions formerly thought to be entirely involuntary, such as heart rate, blood pressure, and blood flow to various parts of the body.

When you visualize certain changes you wish to take place in your body, they tend to occur even though you may be unaware of the underlying mechanisms.

1. Lie on your back. Relax your arms at your sides, palms turned upward. Close your eyes. Relax your jaw and breathe regularly.
2. As you inhale, imagine that you are being breathed into, so that you are the unresisting recipient of breath. Visualize your torso enlarging, and every cell absorbing life-giving properties from the air entering your body.
3. With the outflow of air during exhalation, visualize your body gently contracting, as metabolic waste products are expelled.
4. Fully focus your attention on the pulsating of your abdomen as it rises and falls.
5. Repeat the exercise (steps 2 to 4) for about ten breath cycles (inhalations and exhalations) at first. Increase the number of cycles as you become more familiar and comfortable with the visualization, and as time permits. Totally surrender yourself to the surface on which you are lying, and observe the process as if you were a silent witness.
6. Resume regular breathing. Open your eyes and return to your usual activities.

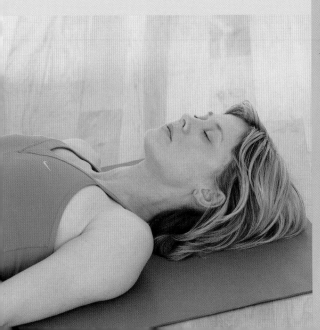

Back and legs: the tree

This pose will help you to achieve perfect balance and will strengthen and tone your back and legs.

NOTES AND SUGGESTIONS
If you focus your attention on a still object in front of you, such as a door handle or a picture on a wall, it will help you to maintain your balance. You can also concentrate on your own rhythmic breathing.

1. Stand tall with your feet close together and parallel to each other. Establish good posture and breathe regularly.
2. Slowly lift one leg and, with the help of your hands, place the sole of the foot against the inner side of your opposite thigh, as high up as is comfortable. Bring your hands together in front of your breastbone. Alternatively, you may stretch your arms sideways at shoulder level, with your wrists relaxed (see right).
3. Stay in this posture for several seconds or as long as you comfortably can. Breathe regularly.
4. When you are ready to come out of the posture, straighten your bent leg and resume your starting position. Relax your hands at your sides.
5. Repeat the exercise, this time balancing on the other foot.
6. Rest briefly.

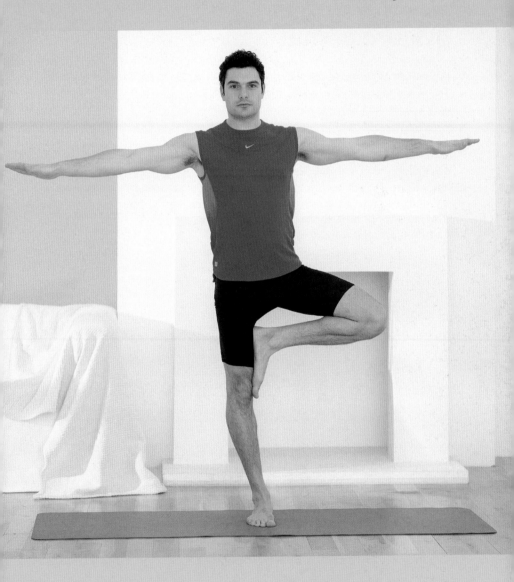

Balance posture

This posture enhances concentration and nerve-muscle coordination. Also called the quadriceps stretch, it conditions the quadriceps muscles at the front of the thighs, which help to straighten the knees.

NOTES AND SUGGESTIONS
When doing this or any other balancing posture, fix your gaze on a still object, such as a door handle, a vase of flowers, or a picture on a wall. It will help you to stay steady. Alternatively, focus your attention on your own slow, regular breathing.

1. Stand tall with your feet comfortably but not too far apart, and your body weight evenly distributed (01). Breathe regularly.
2. Shift your weight on to one foot. Focus your attention on your breathing to help you to stay steady, or on a still object in front of you, such as a door handle.
3. Bend your other leg and point the foot backward, grasp your foot with the hand on the same side,

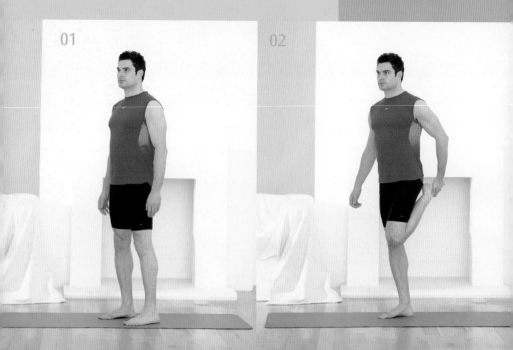

01

02

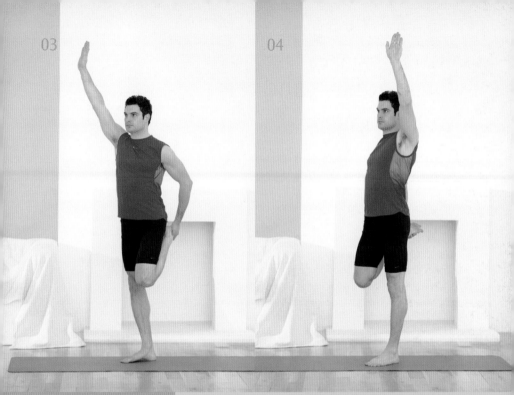

and bring it as close to the buttock on that side as you can with ease (02).

4. Raise your opposite arm straight up (03).

5. Maintain this posture for several seconds or as long as you wish, remembering to breathe regularly.

6. Slowly resume your starting position.

7. Repeat the exercise (steps 2 to 6) on the other side (04).

8. Rest.

When you have gained some mastery of this posture, you may welcome the challenge of a variation: Slowly and carefully bend forward.

Still holding the foot of your bent leg, push it away from your buttocks. Move your body as a unit and keep breathing regularly.

Back, ankles, and feet: squatting

One quarter of the human race habitually take the weight off their feet by squatting. A deep squat position for work and rest is used by millions of people in Africa, Asia, and Latin America.

WHAT IT DOES

Squatting reduces any exaggerated curve of the lower spine, thus lessening tension on spinal muscles and ligaments. It reduces pressure on spinal discs. Consequently, the back is both strengthened and relaxed, and back problems and discomfort are minimized. Squatting is also excellent for strengthening the ankles and feet.

NOTES AND SUGGESTIONS

If you have varicose veins, alternately squat and get up again, several times in succession.

Look for ways to incorporate squatting during daily activities: attending to a small child; dusting the lower parts of furniture; putting in or retrieving something from the lower drawer of a cabinet; weeding.

I also like to practise squatting while waiting for the timer to signal that the evening meal is ready.

1. Stand with your legs comfortably apart. Distribute your body weight evenly between your feet. Breathe regularly.
2. Slowly bend your knees, lowering your buttocks until you are sitting on your heels. Bring your hands together as if in prayer (see right).
3. Stay in this posture for several seconds or as long as you comfortably can.
4. Resume your starting position.

CAUTION
■ *Avoid the squatting posture after the 34th week of pregnancy, until your baby's head is fully engaged, or if you experience pain in the pubic area. Avoid it if you have haemorrhoids or have had a cervical stitch (Shirodkar suture) inserted.*

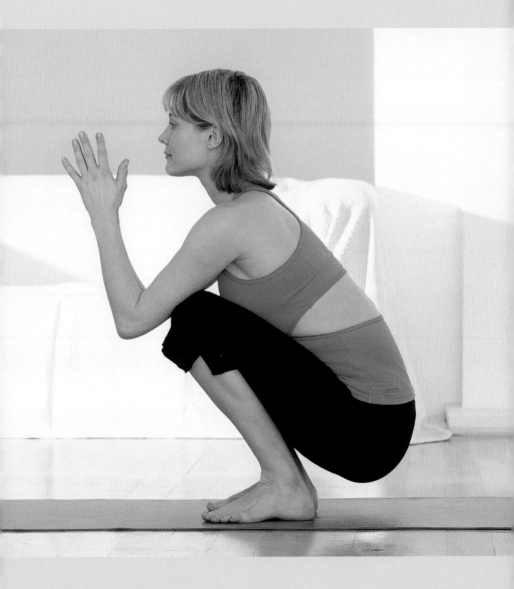

Meditation

Think of meditation as a natural "tool", rather than a mysterious, esoteric practice. It is a device used to relax the conscious mind without clouding awareness. Doctors describe the meditative state as one of "hypometabolic wakefulness", which means that your metabolism has decreased even though you are still awake and conscious. They also refer to it as a state of "restful alertness", an apparent contradiction.

When you are asleep, for instance, your heart rate becomes slower, oxygen consumption decreases, and consciousness fades. When you are awake, by contrast, your heart rate quickens, oxygen consumption increases, and you are usually alert. These opposites are united during meditation so that, although your body becomes deeply relaxed, you are conscious and your mind is clear.

Meditation, then, is a technique for quietening a restless mind and discouraging it from pursuing thoughts and ideas. You focus your attention on one thing or activity to the exclusion of everything else. When the mind is quiet, you feel peaceful. With so many stimuli bombarding your senses every day and competing for our attention, it is no wonder that you might often feel stressed. Meditating regularly provides an antidote since it requires us, for a little while, to distance ourselves from these relentless environmental demands.

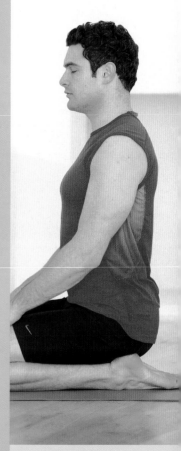

Benefits of meditation

Just as athletes tune and train their bodies, meditation
tunes and trains the mind. For lasting value, it must be
practised regularly. Regular meditation practice helps
to bring deep-seated tensions to the surface so that
you can examine them and attempt to resolve them.
When you confront and deal honestly with unresolved
issues, you begin to be more at ease with yourself and
more comfortable in your relationships with others.
This results in a greater sense of self-worth, more self-
confidence, and better productivity. It also contributes
to increased self-control, so that events and
circumstances that previously seemed insurmountable
now begin to appear manageable. Meditation helps to
integrate and strengthen your personality, allowing
you to become serene and competent.

Long-term meditation helps to decrease metabolic
age. People who meditate regularly visit their doctor
and are admitted to hospital less often than those who
do not meditate routinely. They also have a lower
incidence of heart disease and cancer. Increasingly,
doctors are recommending daily meditation as an
adjunct to treatment for a variety of disorders
including heart disease, high blood pressure,
migraine, stomach and intestinal ulcers, and certain
nervous system conditions. Before starting to practise
meditation, however, check with your doctor.

You can meditate before a public appearance,
interview, or exam, before surgery, or before the
children come home from school – any time, in fact,
that you anticipate a demanding, or stressful situation.

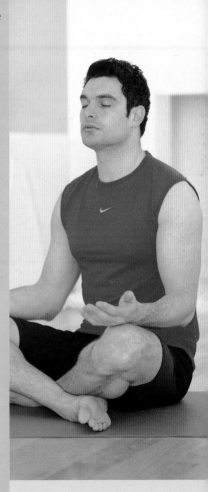

How meditation works

During meditation, oxygen consumption and carbon dioxide elimination both decrease markedly without an alteration in their balance. This means that the circulatory system is functioning efficiently and that the heart's workload is reduced. The heart and respiration rates both decrease, indicating a state of deep relaxation.

Skin resistance increases significantly, denoting a calm emotional state. Metabolic rate drops by about 20 per cent, with a corresponding fall in blood pressure. Lactate ion concentration (thought to affect muscle tone and emotional state) decreases by about 33 per cent. And brainwave recordings on an electro-encephalograph (EEG) show an unusual abundance of alpha waves, signifying that the brain is alert yet wonderfully relaxed.

PREPARING TO MEDITATE
Because it is usually easier to gain control over the body than over the mind, a good way to start preparing for a session of meditation is to do the simple stretching exercises described in Chapter Two, or other similar exercises.

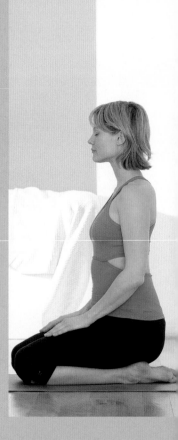

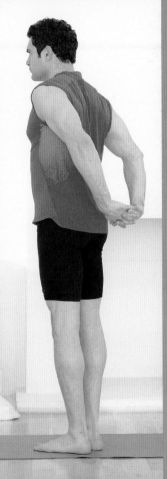

The next preparatory step for meditation is to be able to stay focused. All the exercises in this book will train you to do this, as they require attentiveness to the movements in synchronization with regular breathing. You will also find the balancing exercises such as the tree (see pp.72–3) and the balance posture (see pp.74–5) useful for this purpose.

In addition, doing the breathing exercises will promote the "one-pointedness" that is necessary for successful meditation.

Another prerequisite is the ability to sit still for up to 20 minutes at a time. Folded-leg postures such as the firm posture (see p.85) and the easy pose (see pp.86–7) will provide you with a stable base and enable you to hold your spine in good vertical alignment. If you find, however, that you are unable to sit for any length of time in one of these postures, choose a sitting position in which you are completely comfortable for the duration of the exercise and use a support for your spine if necessary.

Sitting still during meditation is important because the less movement and distraction there is, the steadier your mind will be.

Meditation in action

Meditation is a focusing of attention on one thing or activity at a time, to the exclusion of everything else. You can apply this principle to many everyday tasks and so reap the benefits that regular meditation brings. These include: greater self-confidence, efficiency, and productivity; better health in general and fewer visits to the doctor; slower ageing. When you are able to turn some of your activities into a meditation of sorts, you will find that you are less easily distracted and stressed.

Here's an example of meditation in action, carried out by a friend of mine, as he prepared a tossed green salad. He seemed totally immersed in the process of meticulously cutting up onions and parsley from his kitchen garden; carefully washing and drying green lettuce leaves and breaking them into bite-sized pieces; slicing and dicing red, ripe tomatoes and radishes, and attentively combining all the ingredients before the final tossing with olive oil and vinegar.

My friend once remarked that this was *his* meditation, so absorbed was he in this activity. He added that when he was engaged in making a salad, he was able to shut everything else out of his mind and so found it a very therapeutic exercise. Not surprisingly, his salads are excellent.

Think of the many things you do in the course of the day. Think of which ones you can realistically do with a similar one-pointedness: arranging flowers; listening as a child or other friend speaks; playing tennis. Put this idea of meditation in action into practice and you will be pleasantly surprised at the results.

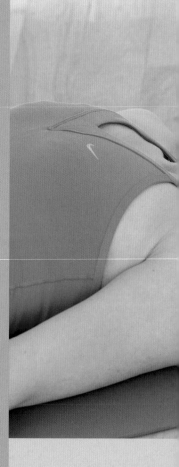

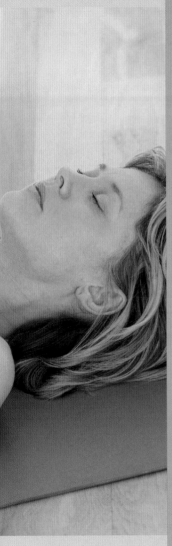

Other guidelines

Daily practice of the pose of tranquillity (see pp.102–7), or any convenient modification of the technique, will train you in the art of relaxing at will, and is therefore well worth your while.

It's best to meditate before rather than after a meal so that the process of digestion doesn't interfere with your concentration.

Choose a quiet place in which to meditate, where you can be assured of at least five minutes of uninterrupted time (to begin with), and about 20 minutes for a longer session. Suitable places include: a quiet room at home or at work; a small empty chapel; a private porch; a garden; beside a pond or lake.

Try to meditate at least once a day; preferably twice. Begin with five minutes per session and gradually increase it to 20 minutes, according to your circumstances and the time available.

If after practising a particular meditation a few times you still do not feel comfortable with it, try another. There's no single way of meditating that is best for everyone. Through experimentation you will find the method that is most compatible with your personality and beliefs. You should always feel better, not worse, after a meditation session.

Be patient and persevere in your meditation. Do not feel disappointed if the expected results are not immediately apparent. The benefits of regular meditation are cumulative, and skill and ease will come with time and repeated practice.

A simple meditation

Meditation is a natural device for relaxing your conscious mind without dulling your awareness. It helps to keep you in the present, as an antidote to apprehension, worry, and depression, which concern past and future events.

NOTES AND SUGGESTIONS

You may substitute any word or short phrase for the word "one" in the exercise on the right. Particularly effective is something related to your religion or other belief system. Suggestions are: "peace", "calm", "serenity"; "love and light"; "I feel calm"; "I am at peace"; "I am free from harm".

When you are faced with, or anticipate a challenging or perplexing situation, try to recall the calm you experienced during or after meditation. Take a few slow breaths, as deep as you can without straining. These simple measures will help to delay your response, so that you will act consciously rather than react impulsively. They will provide you with a focal point to help you to maintain a degree of control. They will assist you in establishing or re-establishing mental equilibrium.

Keep your breathing slow and smooth throughout. If your thoughts wander during your meditation, and they will at first, gently guide them back to both the breathing and the repetition of the word "one" or your chosen phrase. With faithful meditation practice, your thoughts will drift off less often as your ability to remain focused improves. Be patient and persevere.

1. Sit comfortably upright, with the crown of your head uppermost. Relax your hands and the rest of your body (see below). Close your eyes. Relax your jaw and breathe regularly. Inhale slowly and smoothly through your nose.
2. As you exhale slowly and smoothly through your nose, mentally say the word "one".
3. Repeat steps 1 and 2 several times in smooth succession.
4. When you are ready to end your period of meditation, do so slowly: open your eyes and gently stretch or massage your limbs.

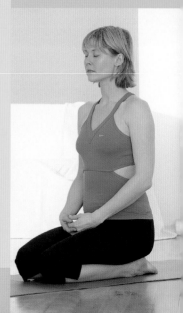

Firm posture

This posture encourages good spinal alignment and therefore healthier functioning of vital structures within the trunk. It is also a useful meditation posture, providing a solid, stable base on which to sit.

NOTES AND SUGGESTIONS

If at first your heels cannot bear your weight, place a cushion between your buttocks and your heels, and stay in this position only briefly. As your knees and ankles become more flexible and your body more conditioned, you will be able to maintain firm posture for a longer time.

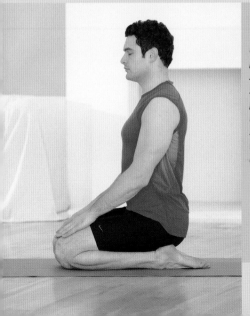

1. Kneel down with your legs together and your body erect but not rigid. Let your feet point straight backward.
2. Slowly lower your body to sit on your heels. Gently place your palms on your knees (see left).
3. Sit tall and breathe regularly. Keep as relaxed as you can.

Easy pose

The easy pose (tailor sitting) provides a stable base and encourages you to hold your spine naturally erect. It promotes relaxation of the back muscles. It brings into play the sartorius, or tailor muscles, which lie across the thighs, from about the front of the hip bones to the shin bones. These are the muscles used in bending the legs and turning them inward.

NOTES AND SUGGESTIONS

You may find it helpful to sit on a cushion or a folded towel or blanket, so that your knees come closer to the floor than they otherwise would.

Because of the firm, stable base this posture provides, it is an excellent one in which to sit for a long period of time, as when meditating or doing breathing exercises. In addition, because easy pose encourages good spinal alignment, it is superb for promoting good posture and related feelings of self-worth and self-confidence.

1. Sit with your legs stretched out in front of you and your hands flat on the floor beside your hips (01).
2. Bend one leg and place the foot of that leg under the opposite thigh (02).
3. Bend the other leg and place the foot under the opposite bent leg (03).
4. Rest your palms gently on your knees or place them upturned, one in the other, in your lap (04).
5. Maintain this posture as long as you comfortably can, breathing regularly and keeping your body relaxed.

CAUTION
■ *Avoid sitting in this or any other folded-legs posture if you experience pain in your pubic area.*

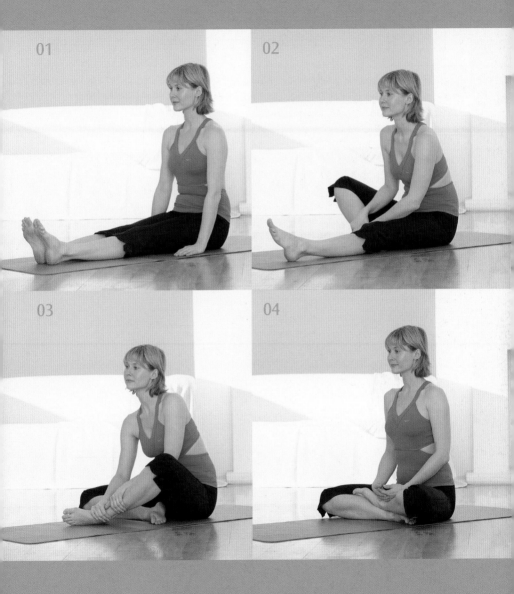

01

02

03

04

Bedtime: preparing for sleep

Sleep experts say that many people who live in industrialized countries are sleep deprived. This is not surprising. Youngsters, for example, get up earlier than they normally would to accommodate the expanding size of many classes at school. They then rush to part-time jobs after their day's studies. In addition, there's homework to do, and sometimes cramming for a test the next day. There are also extra-curricular activities such as soccer, hockey, or track and field practice. All this means going to bed late and being rudely awakened, after perhaps only six hours sleep, by the unwelcome ringing of an alarm clock.

Sleep fulfils two important functions: the restoration of energy and the regulation and resynchronization of the body. Sleep deprivation over time can have serious consequences, among which are low energy and motivation, poor concentration and performance and, in more extreme cases, depression and psychosis.

If lack of sleep has resulted in ill health, please consult a doctor. There are several simple measures you can take to help prevent this, and to promote sound, refreshing sleep. If you cannot immediately add to the number of hours of sleep you are currently obtaining, you can certainly do something about the quality of your sleep. Mild exercise after supper can promote sleep of good quality, whereas more vigorous activity may prove too stimulating. Most of the warm-up exercises in Chapter Two are suitable for evening practice. The breathing exercises (except for the dynamic cleansing breath) are also appropriate.A warm (not hot) bath, in which the water is between

WAKE REFRESHED
Getting a good night's sleep makes all the difference to how you feel throughout each day, so it's worth spending a little time preparing for bedtime to ensure that you get the best quality sleep possible.

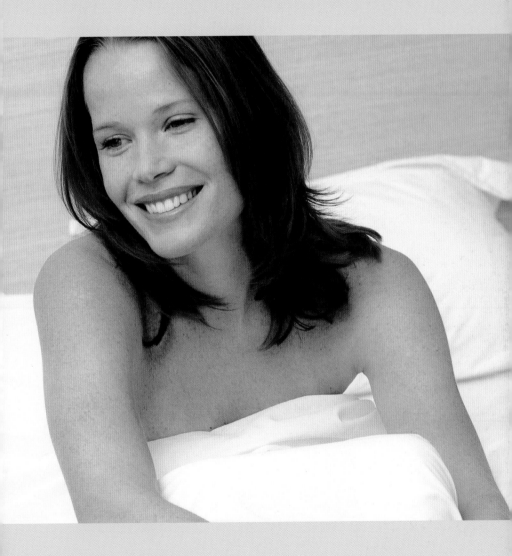

35°C and 38°C (95°F and 100°F) is relaxing, and some people find it sleep-inducing. The addition of an aromatic oil with calming properties, such as bergamot, cedarwood, chamomile, lavender, neroli, or rose, may enhance the mellow mood conducive to sweet sleep.

Just before going to bed, avoid reading material that is highly stimulating or watching television shows which are disturbing or exciting, if you have observed that they prevent you from sleeping soundly.

As you prepare yourself for sleep, turn your thoughts away from unpleasant matters. If possible, try to resolve any misunderstandings or other discord before you finally turn in for the night. Practise the pose of tranquillity (see pp.102–7) or the alternate nostril breathing (see pp.108–9).

Should you experience difficulty falling or staying asleep because of hunger, try eating a light carbohydrate snack before you go to bed.

Consider also taking two or three calcium tablets with warm milk, but first check with your doctor or a qualified nutrition counsellor.

Avoid drinking alcohol or smoking shortly before going to sleep. Alcohol may help you fall asleep, but it will also cause you to have a restless night, leaving you feeling groggy and tired when you wake up. Avoid stimulants such as regular tea, coffee, cocoa, and cola drinks. There are many relaxing herbal teas that are more suitable for drinking at bedtime. Check with your doctor to ensure that the herbal infusion of your choice will not clash with any medication you take.

Make sure that the room where you habitually sleep is sufficiently warm or cool, dark or softly lit, as you prefer, and free of any disturbing noises.

Sleep on a mattress that adequately supports your back without being rigid, keep the bedclothes to the minimum necessary for desired warmth or coolness, use a pillow that gives your head and neck good support, and wear loose, comfortable clothing.

The ten-minute pre-sleep exercise sequence that follows is designed to counteract any tension that you may have accumulated during the day, to promote relaxation, and to set a scene conducive to peaceful sleep. Modify the sequence to suit your own special needs. You can do so by reducing or increasing the number of repetitions, for example, or by increasing or decreasing the "holding" period during which you maintain a particular stretch or posture.

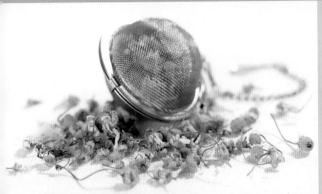

A BEDTIME DRINK

To aid a restful night, drink a herbal tea made with catmint, chamomile flowers, dill, lime blossom, passion flowers, or valerian, all of which induce a pleasant drowsiness. Please check with your doctor that the herbal tea of your choice will not react with any medication you are taking.

Ten-minute evening sequence

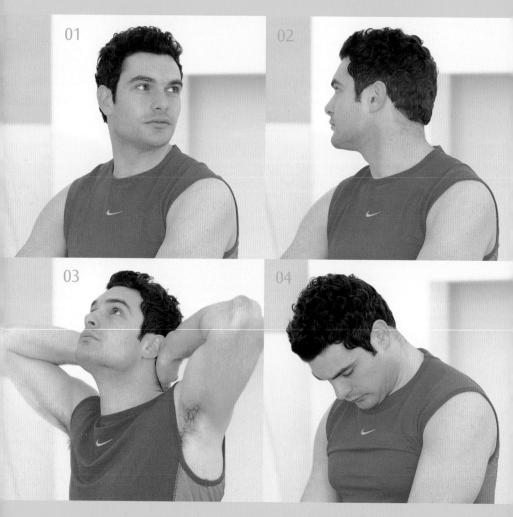

05

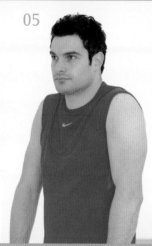

06

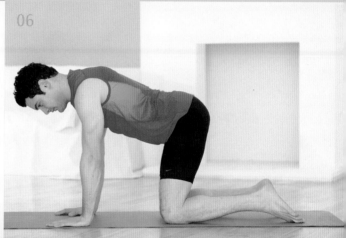

■ *Neck stretches (see pp.18–19) 3 to 5 times in each direction (01–04).*
■ *Shoulder exercises (see pp.22–23) 3 to 5 times each (05).*
■ *Ankle rotation (see p.32) 3 to 5 times in each direction.*
■ *Pelvic tilt on all fours (see p.96) 3 to 5 times (06, 07).*

07

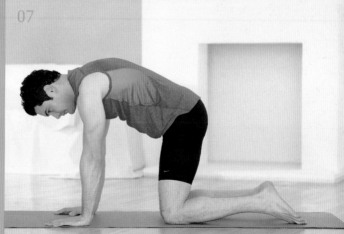

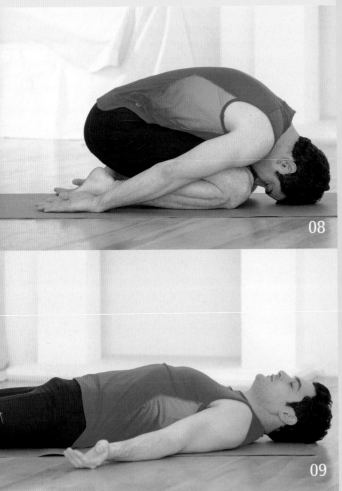

■ *Afterward, rest in the curling leaf posture (see p.97) (08).*
■ *Then do the half shoulderstand (see pp.98–9) or full shoulderstand (see pp.100–1). Maintain the posture for 20 to 60 seconds or more. Alternatively, you can do the legs-up posture (see p.70).*
■ *For recovery do the pose of tranquillity (see pp.102–7) (09, 10) or alternate nostril breathing (see pp.108–9) for the time remaining, or lie in the legs-up posture (see p.70) (11) and practise all-body breathing (see p.71), or indeed any other breathing exercise of your choice (except the dynamic cleansing breath).*

08

09

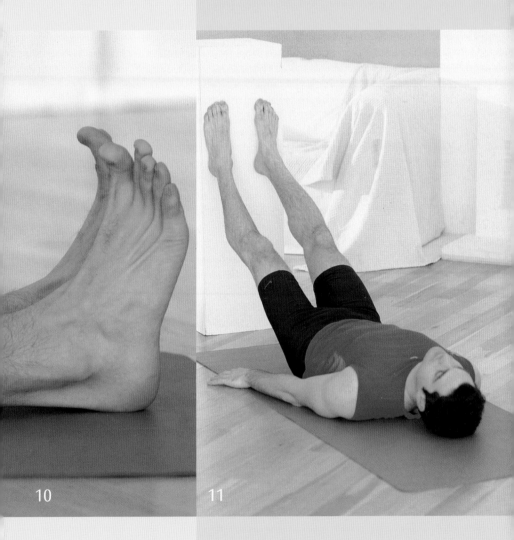

10

11

Pelvic tilt on all fours

Pelvic tilting helps to keep your spine flexible. It conditions the back muscles which support your spine, and tones and firms your abdominal muscles, which complement your back muscles as spinal supports.

1. Get on your hands and knees in the all fours position (01).
2. Exhaling, lower your head, tuck your hips down, and arch your shoulders, so that your entire back is rounded (02). Concentrate on the tilting of the pelvis rather than on the arching of the shoulders.
3. Inhale and resume your starting position.
4. Repeat steps 2 and 3 several times in smooth succession.
5. Rest.

Curling leaf

This posture, which is also called the pose of a child, helps to keep your spine flexible. As you breathe regularly while maintaining the completed posture, your internal organs receive a gentle, therapeutic massage which promotes circulation and facilitates elimination. Curling leaf is also a very relaxing posture and an excellent one to practise following backward-bending exercises.

NOTES AND SUGGESTIONS
If you cannot get your head down on to the mat, place a cushion, pillow, or folded towel in front of you, and rest your forehead on it.

1. Sit on your heels, as in the firm posture. Relax your jaw and breathe regularly (01).
2. Bend forward slowly, and rest your forehead on the mat; or turn your face to the side. Relax your arms and hands beside you (02).
Stay in this posture for several seconds or for as long as you feel comfortable in it, breathing regularly.
3. Slowly resume your starting position.

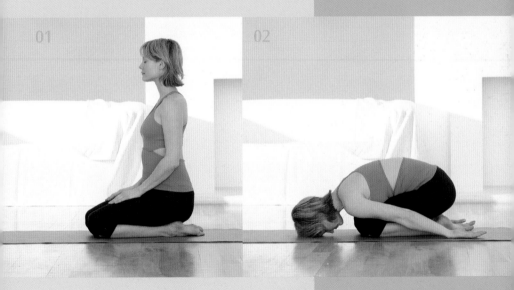

Half shoulderstand

The health-giving benefits of this inverted posture are the result of the stretching and contraction of three muscle groups: your back muscles which are stretched, your abdominal muscles which are contracted, and the muscles at the front of your neck which are also contracted. The organs within your torso are revitalized, thereby improving circulation and also the function of the endocrine glands and the nervous system. By summoning the aid of gravitational forces, moreover, the half shoulderstand (and other inverted postures) promotes circulation to the upper body, including the face and scalp, and so enriches those tissues.

CAUTIONS
- *Avoid this and other inverted postures if you have an eye or ear disorder, or if you suffer from heart disease, high blood pressure or other circulatory abnormality.*
- *Do not practise inverted postures while you are menstruating.*
- *Check with your doctor before attempting to do the half shoulderstand or other head-low, hips-high postures.*

01

02

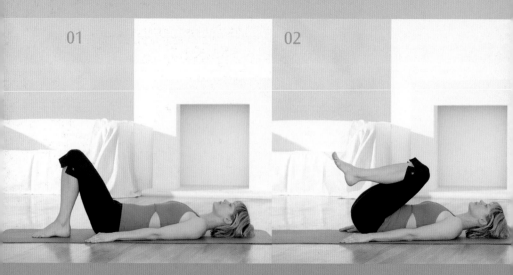

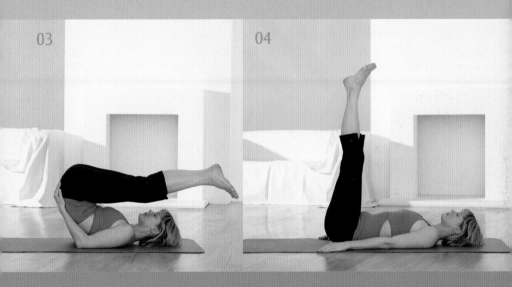

1. *Lie on your back. Bend your knees and rest the soles of your feet flat on the mat (01). Keep your arms close to your sides. Breathe regularly throughout the exercise.*
2. *Bring first one knee, then the other, to your chest (02).*
3. *Straighten one leg at a time until your feet are pointing upward.*
4. *Kick backward with both feet at once, until your hips are off the mat. Support your hips with your hands, thumbs in front (03).*
5. *Maintain this posture for a few seconds to begin with; longer as you become more comfortable with it.*
6. *To come out of the posture, rest your hands on the mat, close to your body. Keep your head firmly pressed to the mat (perhaps tilting your chin slightly upward), and slowly and carefully lower your torso, from top to bottom, on to the mat (04). Bend your knees and stretch out your legs, one at a time.*
7. *Rest.*

Full shoulderstand

The benefits derived from the full shoulderstand are the same as those of the half shoulderstand (see pp.98–9). In addition, the full shoulderstand enhances thyroid gland function: the thyroid gland controls your body's metabolism, so that when it is functioning well all cells and tissues benefit.

1. Lie on your back. Bend your knees and rest the soles of your feet flat on the mat. Keep your arms close to your sides. Breathe regularly throughout the exercise.
2. Bring first one knee, then the other, to your chest.

CAUTIONS
■ *These are the same as for the half shoulderstand (see pp.98–9).*
■ *Avoid doing the full shoulderstand if you suffer from neck pain.*
■ *If you suffer from cramp, keep your feet flat in the shoulderstand, rather than pointing them.*

01

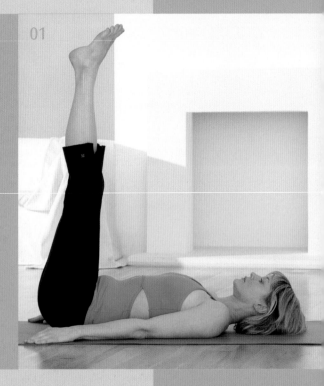

02

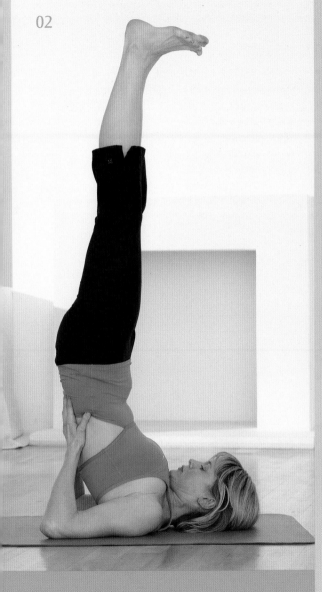

3. Straighten one leg at a time until your feet are pointing upward (01).

4. Kick back with both feet at once, until your hips are off the mat. Support your hips with your hands, with your thumbs in front.

5. Gradually move your hands, one at a time, toward your upper back, until your body is in as vertical a position as you can manage with complete comfort. Your chin should then come in contact with your chest, and your whole body should be as relaxed as possible (02).

6. Maintain this posture for a few seconds to begin with, working up to a minute or more as you become more comfortable with it.

7. To come out of the posture, tilt your feet slightly backward. Rest your arms beside your body and keep your head pressed to the mat. Slowly lower your hips to the mat. Bend your legs at the knees and lower them slowly, one at a time, on to the mat.

8. Rest.

Pose of tranquillity

This is a splendid exercise for helping to combat many forms of stress. Practised in the evening after a day of intense work, it is excellent for inducing sound, refreshing sleep. It is also very useful in the management of pain and anxiety states, and for counteracting fatigue and promoting calm.

Regular practice of the technique also helps to keep blood pressure within the normal range, and it is, in addition, a beneficial complement to treatments for heart disorders and peptic ulcers.

RECORD YOUR VOICE
If it makes it easier for you, you can record the instructions for the pose of tranquillity using a tape-recorder. Speak slowly and soothingly, or ask a friend with a clear, pleasing voice to do so for you. Listen to the recording as the need arises.

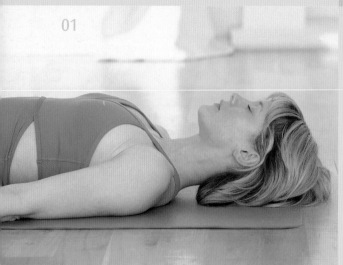

01

1. Lie on your back with your legs comfortably separated and stretched out in front of you. Relax your arms at your sides, a little away from your body, with your palms upturned. Position your head for maximum comfort and close your eyes. Relax your jaw and breathe regularly (01). This is the basic position. Suggestions for variations are given in the Notes and Suggestions (see p.103).

NOTES AND SUGGESTIONS

You may practise the pose of tranquillity in bed, if you are unwell, for instance; or in a reclining chair that gives adequate support to your neck and back. Modify the exercise instructions accordingly. You may also practise it while lying on your back, with your knees bent and your lower legs resting on a padded chair. Or you may practise it in the legs-up posture (see p.70).

Use whatever props and aids you need to provide good support for your body, particularly your neck and lower back, so that you are very comfortable. Suitable props include rolled or folded towels, folded blankets, pillows, or cushions.

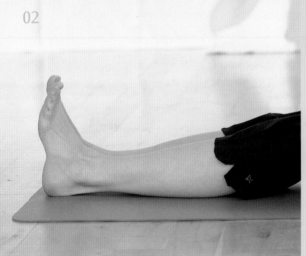

02

2. Push your heels away, bringing your toes toward you (02). Note the resulting stiffness in your legs. Maintain this tension for a few seconds, but continue to breathe regularly. (This maintaining of tension will be referred to as "hold" from now on.)
3. Let go of the stiffness. Relax your knees, legs, ankles, feet, and toes. (This letting go of tension will be referred to as "release" from now on.) Let your legs sink with their full weight on to the mat.

Keep a sweater or blanket and a pair of warm socks nearby. Use them to prevent you becoming cold as your body cools down during relaxation.

Loosely tie a scarf around your eyes, or wear a pair of eye-shades to hasten relaxation by the complete exclusion of light.

In step 13 of the exercise instructions (see p.106), use imagery with which you feel most comfortable. You may, for example, visualize yourself lying on a warm, sandy beach while a gentle breeze caresses your face, arms, and legs. Each time you breathe in, imagine the surf rolling toward your feet, bringing peace and rejuvenating properties with it. Each time you breathe out, imagine the surf rolling out again, taking with it the cares, concerns, and weariness of the day.

Practise the pose of tranquillity any time you need to recharge and re-energize yourself, such as after an especially demanding day or a particularly trying experience that has left you feeling drained. Practise it when you feel anxiety mounting and when you long for a sense of calm and well-being.

Do this relaxation technique in a quiet place where you can be sure of 10 to 20 minutes on your own without interruption.

When you are well versed in the technique, you can dispense with alternately tightening and relaxing muscle groups and so reduce the time required to practise it. For example, while focusing attention on your feet, mentally say: "Feet, let go of your tightness. Relax." Then consciously relax them. Work from the feet up, and remember to include the facial muscles.

4. Tighten your buttocks. Hold. Release. Relax your hips. On exhalation, press the small of your back (waist) firmly toward the mat. Feel your abdominal muscles tighten. Hold the tightness as long as your exhalation lasts. Release the tension as you inhale. Breathe regularly. Relax your back and abdomen. (This is a lying version of the pelvic tilt earlier in this chapter (pp.60–1)).
5. Inhale and squeeze your shoulder blades together. Release as you exhale. Relax your shoulders and upper back. Breathe regularly.
6. Shrug your shoulders as if trying to touch your ears with them (03). Relax your shoulders on release.
7. Carefully tilt your head slightly backward. Feel the gentle stretch of your neck (04). Carefully re-position your head for maximum comfort. Relax your throat.
8. Carefully tilt your head forward, tucking in your chin (05). Hold. Release to neutral position. Relax your neck.

03

04

05

9. *Raise your eyebrows and wrinkle your forehead (06). Hold. Release. Relax your forehead. Relax your scalp muscle, which goes from just above the eyebrows to the back of the head.*
10. *Squeeze your eyes shut tightly. Hold. Release. Relax your eyes.*
11. *Exhaling, open your mouth wide. Stick out your tongue as far as you comfortably can (07). Open your eyes wide, as if staring. Feel all your facial muscles tighten. (This is the lion pose, which can be done as a separate exercise to reduce facial tension.) Hold the tension as long as your exhalation lasts. Inhale and pull in your tongue. Close your mouth and eyes. Relax your jaw, tongue, lips, throat, and facial muscles. Breathe regularly.*
12. *Stiffen and raise your arms. Make tight fists (08). Hold. Release. Relax your arms and hands. Let them sink heavily on to the mat.*
13. *Now give your full attention to your breathing. As you inhale slowly and as*

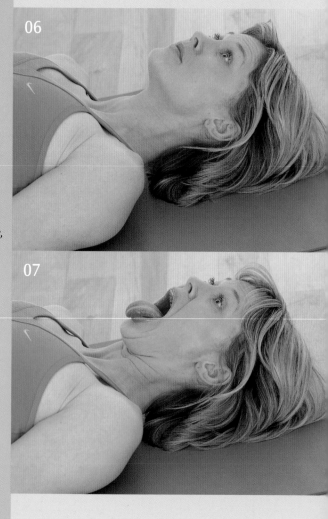

06

07

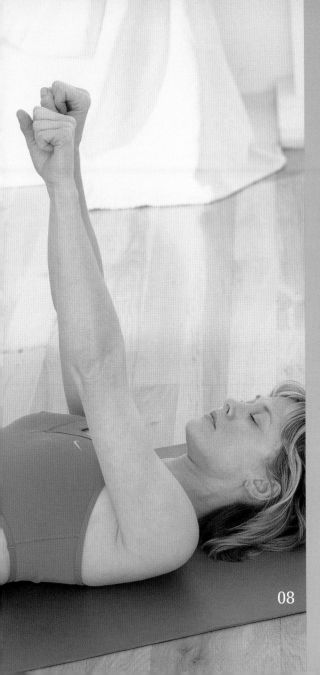

deeply as you can without strain, visualize filling your system not only with health-giving oxygen, but also with positive forces such as love, hope, joy, and calm. As you exhale smoothly without force, visualize eliminating from your body not only wastes such as carbon dioxide, but also negative influences such as sadness, resentment, anxiety, and hopelessness. Each time you exhale, let your body sink a little more into the mat, until every trace of residual tension has vanished.

14. When you feel ready to end your session of deep relaxation, do so slowly and with awareness: make small, gentle movements, such as wriggling your toes and fingers, or rolling your head from side to side. You may also, if you wish, gently massage parts of your body. When ready to sit up, roll on to your side and use your hands to help you. Do not come straight up from a supine position, as this may put a strain your back. Never get up suddenly.

08

Alternate nostril breathing

This exercise stimulates the inner lining of the nose by altering the air flow and sending sequential impulses to the two hemispheres of the brain.

Alternate nostril breathing helps to integrate the functioning of these two hemispheres. The results include a harmonizing of mind and body, and greater mental and physical energy when this is needed.

This is a very soothing exercise that helps to counteract anxiety, which can aggravate pain and other discomforts. It is, in addition, a useful antidote for sleeplessness.

NOTES AND SUGGESTIONS

You may try alternate nostril breathing while standing, or even while lying down.

With your eyes open, you can try this exercise (and most of the other breathing exercises in this book) in a variety of places, including school, your bedside, at your desk or computer, filing cabinet, photocopier, or fax machine (if you can do so unobserved), while waiting to pick up a child from school, in a parked car, during television advertising breaks. Look out for opportunities and modify the exercises to suit yourself.

1. Sit or stand tall and observe good posture. Relax your body, relax your jaw, and breathe regularly.
2. Rest your left hand in your lap, on your thigh or knee, or on the arm rest of a chair.
3. Arrange the fingers of your right hand as follows: fold the two middle fingers toward your palm (or rest them lightly on the bridge of your nose). Use your thumb on your right nostril, once the exercise is in progress, and your ring finger (or ring and little fingers) on your left nostril (01).
4. Close your eyes and begin. Close your right nostril and inhale slowly, smoothly, and as deeply as you can without strain, through your left nostril (02).

01

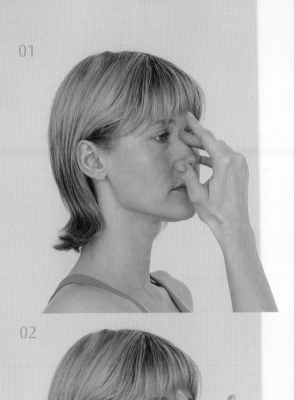

02

5. *Close your left nostril and release the closure of your right nostril. Exhale.*
6. *Inhale slowly and deeply through your right nostril.*
7. *Close your right nostril and release the closure of your left nostril. Exhale. This completes one "round" of alternate nostril breathing.*
8. *Repeat steps 4 to 7 in smooth succession as many times as you wish, until you begin to feel a sense of calm.*
9. *Relax your right arm and hand. Resume regular breathing. Open your eyes.*

Weekend yoga programme

The yoga exercises that you have been incorporating into your daily schedule throughout the week will have trained and conditioned your body and mind in a slow and gentle way, in readiness for a longer weekend workout. Here is a sample programme, which you can modify to suit your own unique requirements. It lasts from 30 minutes to one hour.

The postures and other exercises in this specimen workout have been carefully selected to: warm up your body; provide arm and leg stretches; exercise your spine backward, forward, and sideways, and also give it gentle torsion (twisting); tone and firm the four sets of abdominal muscles that form what is known as the "abdominal corset", and which contribute to spinal health. The programme includes, in addition, an inverted posture to help counteract the effects of the constant downward pull of gravity, and breathing, concentration, visualization, meditation, and relaxation techniques to assist you in regaining a sense of calm and control.

The exercises are arranged so as to allow for a smooth transition from one to the other, but you can vary their order as you wish.
- *Neck stretches (see pp.18–19) 3 to 5 times in each direction (01).*
- *Butterfly (see pp.28–9) 15 to 30 times (02).*
- *Lying twist (see pp.26–7) 5 to 8 times in each direction (03).*
- *Sun salutations (see pp.33–7) 2 to 6 sets (04): 2 to 6 sets.*

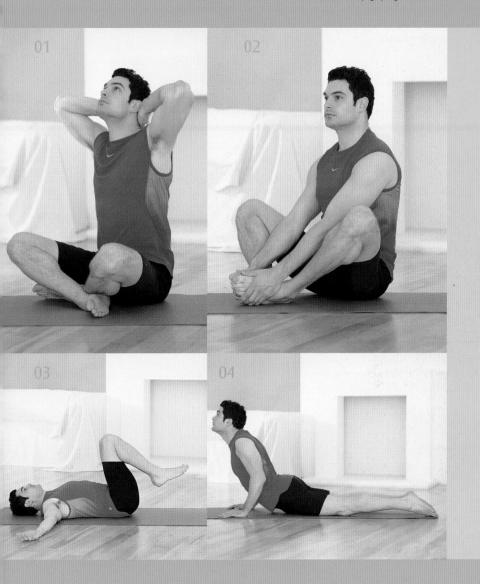

■ *Half moon (see p.116) (05).*
■ *Tree (see pp.72–3) (06)*
or balance posture (see
pp.74–5).
■ *Spinal twist (see*
pp.118–19) (07).
■ *Yoga sit-up (see p.120) (08).*

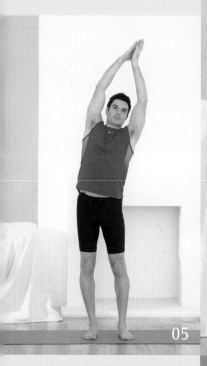

05

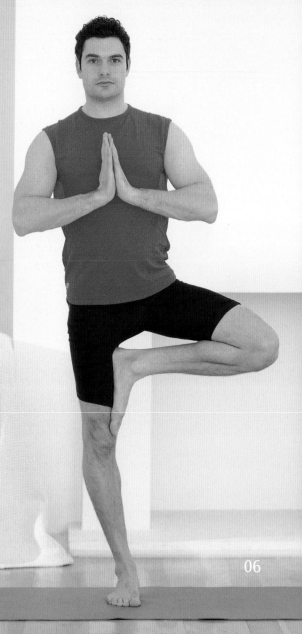

06

07

08

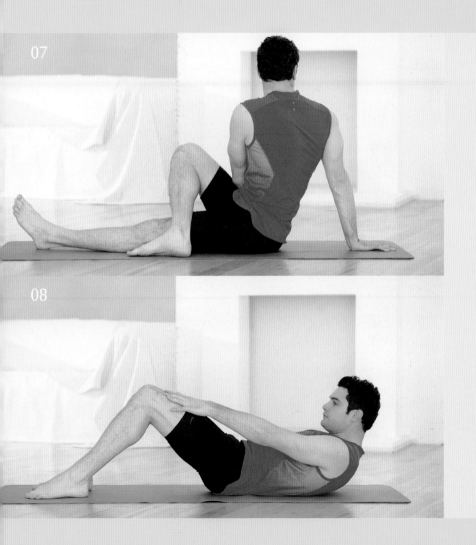

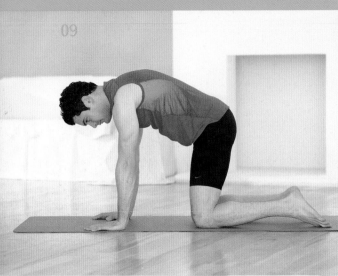

■ *Pelvic tilt on all fours (see p.96) (09), followed by the bridge (see p.117) (10).*
■ *Half shoulderstand (see pp.98–9) or full shoulder-stand (see pp.100–1) (11).*
■ *Breathing exercise of your choice (12).*
■ *The humming breath (see p.121) or other meditation of your choice (13).*
■ *Step 1 of the pose of tranquillity (see p.102) (14).*

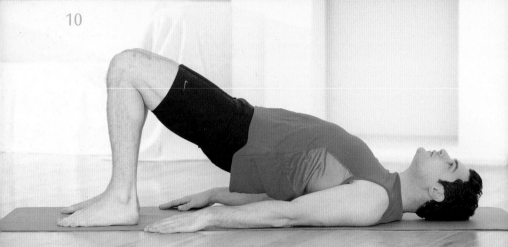

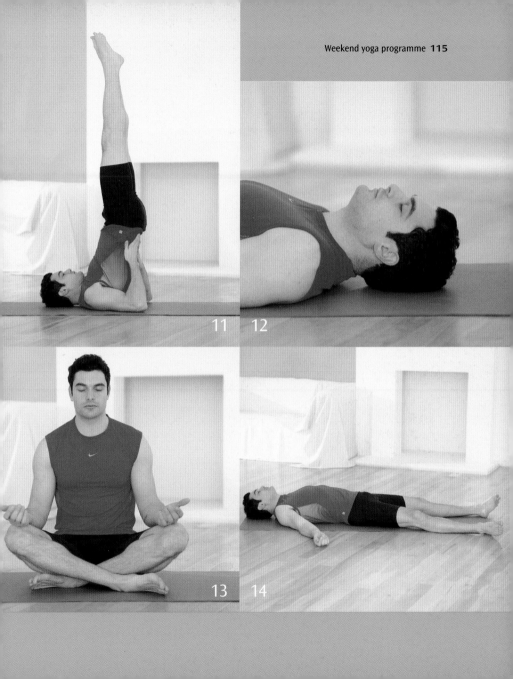

11

12

13

14

Half moon

The half moon gives a lateral (sideways) stretch to your torso, and so contributes to the health of your spine. It also helps to keep your shoulder joints flexible and it exercises the midriff to discourage a build-up of fat. In addition, it facilitates deep breathing.

NOTES AND SUGGESTIONS
In step 2, keep your arms alongside your ears, so that when you bend it will be a true sideways bend rather than a forward bend.

1. Stand naturally erect, with your feet close together and your body weight evenly distributed between them. Relax your jaw and breathe regularly.
2. On an inhalation, bring your arms upward, pressing your palms together if you can (01).
3. As you exhale, slowly and carefully bend your body to one side to form a graceful sideways arch (02).
4. Hold the posture for several seconds or as long as you comfortably can while breathing regularly.
5. Inhale and bring your arms back to the upright position. Exhale and lower your arms to your sides.
6. Repeat the exercise on the other side.
7. Rest.

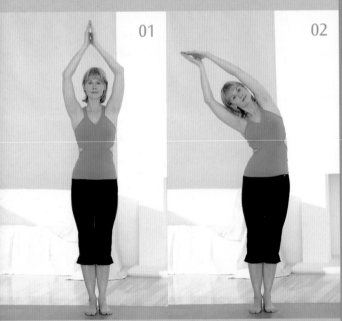

01   02

Bridge

Excellent for toning the back and abdominal muscles, the bridge also helps to keep your spine strong and flexible, and gives your body a therapeutic stretch.

NOTES AND SUGGESTIONS
Combine with the lying pelvic tilt (p.104). Do the pelvic tilt first, then move smoothly into the bridge. Or try this variation: fully stretch your arms and fingers overhead and point your knees as far from your body as you comfortably can.

1. Lie on your back with your legs bent and the soles of your feet flat on the mat, comfortably close to your buttocks. Relax your arms close to your sides, with your palms turned downward. Relax your jaw and breathe regularly.
2. Inhaling, raise your hips, then slowly and smoothly raise the rest of your back until your torso is fully raised (see left). Remember to keep your arms and hands pressed to the mat.
3. Hold the posture for as long as you are comfortable in it, while continuing to breathe regularly.
4. Slowly and smoothly lower your torso in reverse motion, from top to bottom, as if curling your spine one bone at a time on to the mat. Synchronize regular breathing with this movement. Stretch out your legs, turn your palms upward, and rest.

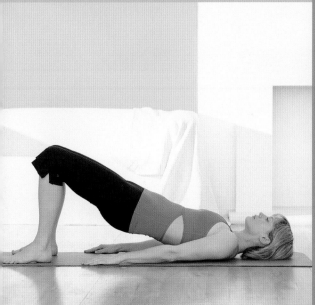

Spinal twist

This is the only yoga posture that requires maximum torsion (twisting) of the spine, first to one side then to the other, causing the vertebrae to rotate one over the other and, at the same time, to bend to the right or left. This spinal action gives a therapeutic massage to nerves branching off the spinal column. The muscles of the lower back are also stretched and contracted during the exercise. This enhances the blood circulation in the area of your kidneys and revitalizes your adrenal glands (located on top of the kidneys).

1. Sit naturally erect on the mat, with your legs stretched out in front of you. Relax your jaw and breathe regularly (01).
2. Bend your left leg at the knee and place your left foot beside the outer side of your right knee (02).
3. Exhaling, slowly and smoothly twist your body to the left and rest both hands on the mat on your left side. Turn your head to look over your left shoulder (03).

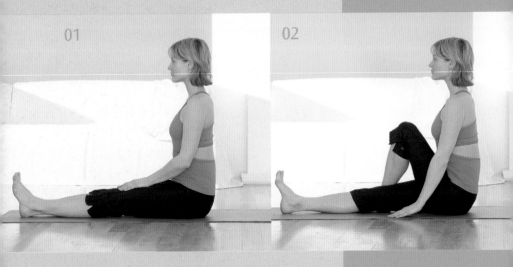

01

02

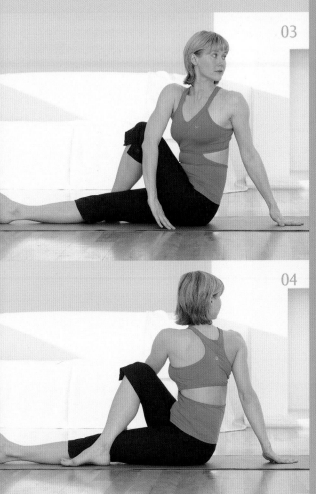

03

04

4. Hold the posture for several seconds or as long as you can with absolute comfort. Keep breathing regularly.
5. Slowly untwist and return to your starting position.
6. Rest briefly.
Repeat the twist on the right side, as follows:
1. Stretch out your left leg in front of you.
2. Bend your right leg at the knee and place your right foot beside the outer side of your left knee.
3. As you exhale, slowly and carefully twist your body to the right and place both hands on the mat at your right side. Turn your head and look over your right shoulder (04).
4. Hold the posture for several seconds or as long as you can with absolute comfort. Continue to breathe regularly.
5. Slowly untwist and return to your starting position.
6. Rest.

Yoga sit-up

Safer to do than the conventional sit-up, the yoga sit-up is superb for developing and maintaining the strength of the abdominal muscles. Strong abdominal muscles help to support the back muscles, and so contribute to the health of the spine.

1. Lie on your back with your legs stretched out in front of you and slightly separated. Relax your arms at your sides. Relax your jaw and breathe regularly.

2. Bend your knees and slide your feet toward your buttocks until the soles are flat on the mat. (Maintain this distance between the feet and buttocks as you practise the sit-up.) Rest your palms on your thighs (01).

3. Exhale as you slowly and carefully raise your head. Keep your gaze on your hands as you slide them along your thighs, as if to touch your knees (02).

4. When you have reached the maximum tolerable tension in your abdomen, stop and hold the posture for a few seconds, or as long as you comfortably can. Keep breathing regularly.

5. Inhale and resume your starting position by slowly curling your spine back on to the mat. Relax your arms and hands at your sides and rest.

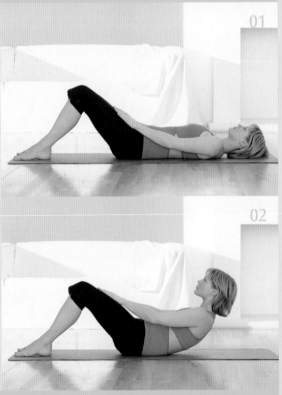

01

02

Humming breath

Sounds can have a powerful effect on the mind. Military music on the battlefield or chants by cheerleaders, for example, tend to excite or agitate people or make them feel aggressive. Other sounds, such as those of a waterfall or a lullaby can promote relaxation and a sense of tranquillity.

One time-honoured way of focusing the mind is to meditate on the repetition of a selected sound. Choose one with which you are comfortable, and which is compatible with your belief system.

The most basic sound is that produced by humming. According to meditation tradition, all sounds are derived from this. It is a very peaceful sound. Interestingly, it is found, with variations, in almost every culture and religious tradition, as part of prayer or meditative ritual. In some instances, the words containing this sound mean "peace" when translated literally: for example "shalom" in Hebrew and "salaam" in Arabic. Repetition of the sound focuses your awareness and promotes a peaceful state.

NOTES AND SUGGESTIONS

Practise the humming breath after a busy or demanding day to help you to regain perspective and a feeling of self-control. Practise it when you feel troubled, to relax and comfort you. Give your complete attention to the breathing and the sound. This pulls your thoughts away from disturbing stimuli.

1. Sit upright with the crown of your head uppermost. Relax your hands. Close your eyes. Relax your jaw and breathe regularly through your nose.

2. Inhale slowly, smoothly, and as deeply as you can without strain.

3. As you exhale slowly and smoothly, make a humming sound, like that of a bee. Let the humming last as long as your exhalation does.

4. Repeat steps 2 and 3 in smooth succession, as many times as you wish, until you feel calm and relaxed.

5. Resume regular breathing. Open your eyes.

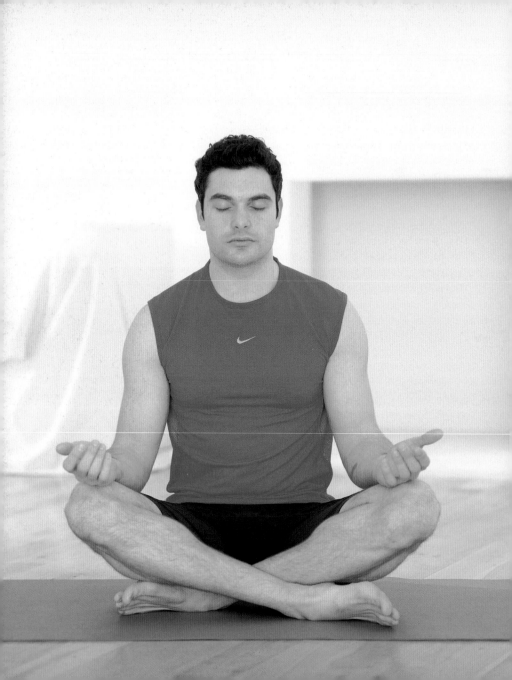

Further reading

Benson, Herbert
The Relaxation Response
William Morrow, 1975

Feuerstein, Georg, Ph.D.
The Yoga Tradition
Hohm Press, 1998

Haynes, Marion E.
Personal Time Management (3rd ed.)
Crisp Learning, 2001

LeShan, Lawrence
How to Meditate
Turnstone Press, 1983

Monro, Dr Robin, Nagarathna, Dr R.,
and Nagendra, Dr H.R.
Yoga for Common Ailments
Gaia Books, 1990

Moyers, Bill
Healing and the Mind
Doubleday, 1993

Rama, Swami, Ballentine, Rudolph, M.D.,
and Hymes, Alan, M.D.
Science of Breath
The Himalayan International Institute of
Yoga Science and Philosophy, 1979

Stroebel, Charles F., M.D.
QR The Quieting Reflex
G.Putnam's Sons, 1982

Weil, Andrew, M.D.
Ask Dr. Weil
The Ballantine Publishing Group, 1998

Weil, Andrew, M.D.
Spontaneous Healing
Alfred A. Knopf, 1995

Weller, Stella
Good Housekeeping Complete Yoga
HarperCollins Illustrated, 2001

Weller, Stella
The Yoga Back Book (rev. ed.)
Thorsons, 2000

Weller, Stella
Well Being for Women
Godsfield Press and Sterling, 1999

Weller, Stella
Yoga Therapy
Thorsons, 1995

Index

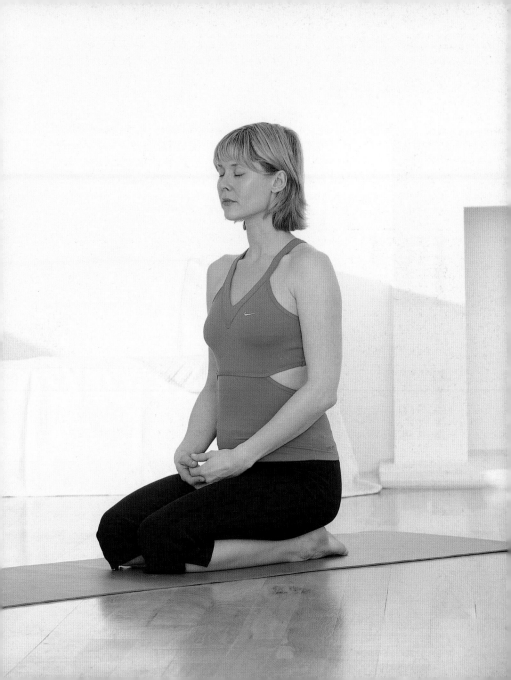

Acknowledgements

Author's dedication

To Gundel, with much love and gratitude.

Author's acknowledgements

Many thanks to everyone who has contributed to this book. I am particularly grateful to Joss Pearson, Gerardine Munroe, Patrick Nugent, Pip Morgan, and the editorial and sales staff at Gaia Books. Thanks also to Michael Whitehead and Warrick Sears of Bridgewater Books, Fiona Biggs, Mike Hemsley, Adam Clement, and Rebecca Barkans.

Special thanks go to David for sharing his expertise in computer skills, and to Walter and Karl for their unfailing support.

Cautions

Care is needed when treating the very young, the elderly, and those suffering from bone problems, epilepsy, clinical depression, cancer, low or high blood pressure, or who are pregnant.

Personal details

Stella Weller is a master of Hatha Yoga and a published author for more than 20 years, specialising in yoga and other health-related subjects. She has more than 12 books in print, some translated into as many as ten languages.

Stella lives in Vancouver, Canada, where she has worked as a Registered Nurse for more than fifteen years. She teaches people how to integrate yoga into their lives, especially those suffering from anxiety and other stress-related disorders.